Cost-Benefit and Cost-Effectiveness Analysis in Policymaking: Cimetidine as a Model

Cost-Benefit and Cost-Effectiveness Analysis in Policymaking: Cimetidine as a Model

Bernard S. Bloom, Ph.D., Editor

**Proceedings of an International Symposium
November 22-24, 1981
Tarpon Springs, Florida**

Sponsored by the Leonard Davis Institute of Health Economics
Center for Health Policy and Planning
University of Pennsylvania

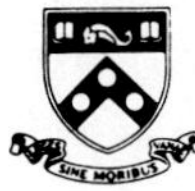

Funded by a Grant from Smith Kline & French Laboratories

Printed in the United States of America
International Standard Book Number :0-935404-58-9
Library of Congress Catalog Card Number : 82-071637

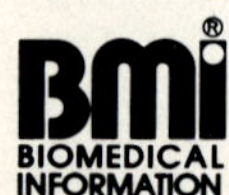

Biomedical Information Corporation Publications
800 Second Avenue
New York, N.Y. 10017

NOTE: Contents of these proceedings are the sole responsibility of the authors and
participants and not of Biomedical Information Corporation, the Leonard Davis
Institute of Health Economics, or Smith Kline & French Laboratories.

Table of Contents

PREFACE

Bernard S. Bloom, Ph.D.

Chief, Health Services Research, Veterans Administration Medical Center
Research Associate Professor, Department of Research Medicine, University of Pennsylvania Medical School
Senior Fellow, Leonard Davis Institute of Health Economics
Philadelphia, Pennsylvania

The development and implementation of rational policies is a major concern of decision makers. Understanding this process is not only an academic problem; for those faced with formulating policies acceptable in a political environment, a practical resolution must be considered. Numerous techniques are available to assist policymakers in devising rational decisions that can be implemented. At the same time, a variety of problems consistently intervene to retard such progress. To understand this problem, the Leonard Davis Institute of Health Economics* of the University of Pennsylvania and Smith Kline & French Laboratories jointly conceived a symposium on the problem of rational policymaking.

Biomedical Information Corporation became responsible for all symposium logistics and published the proceedings. A National Advisory Committee was formed to assist in planning, designing, and developing the symposium. Committee members, representing policymakers and academic researchers from diverse backgrounds, were:

Chairman
William P. Pierskalla, Ph.D., Director
Leonard Davis Institute of Health Economics
University of Pennsylvania
Philadelphia, Pennsylvania

Clifton A. Cole, M.P.A.
Chief Deputy Director
Medical Care Services
Department of Health Services
Sacramento, California

James T. Doluisio, Ph.D.
Dean, College of Pharmacy
University of Texas
Austin, Texas

Harvey V. Fineberg, M.D., Ph.D.
Professor of Health Policy and Management
Center for the Analysis of
Health Practices
Harvard School of Public Health
Boston, Massachusetts

Myrle A. Myers, R.Ph., M.S.
Chief, Pharmacy and Ambulatory Care Service
Division of Medical Assistance
Department of Social Services
Denver, Colorado

Duncan Neuhauser, Ph.D.
Professor
Department of Epidemiology
and Community Health
School of Medicine
Case Western Reserve University
Cleveland, Ohio

Paul D. Stolley, M.D.
Professor
Department of Medicine, Section
of General Medicine
University of Pennsylvania
Philadelphia, Pennsylvania

The symposium was held November 22-24, 1981 in Tarpon Springs, Florida. Special appreciation is due to Ronald Stewart and Morton Paterson, Ph.D., of Smith Kline & French Laboratories for their advice and assistance. From Biomedical Information, Mr. Gerald Diamond provided important advice; Ms. Ronnie Goldstein was responsible for all symposium logistics, and Ms. Betty Treiber was the managing editor of the symposium proceedings. Ms. Joanne Levy of the Leonard Davis Institute of Health Economics served as the overall project manager and provided the guidance and organizational assistance required for the success of the symposium. Ms. Jennifer Conway ably assisted in preparing the symposium proceedings.

---

* The Leonard Davis Institute of Health Economics is an interdisciplinary center for research and education in the organization, financing and delivery of health care. It is a joint enterprise of the School of Medicine, School of Dental Medicine and Wharton School of the University of Pennsylvania. Established in 1967, the Institute enables University faculty and staff to work together on issues of concern in management and policy.

INTRODUCTION

Background, Goals and Objectives, Forum

Background, Goals and Objectives, Forum

Bernard S. Bloom, Ph.D.

BACKGROUND

In their quest for rational decisions, policymakers are frequently faced with a variety of problems. Often, the single overwhelming concern is the amount and type of information needed in order to determine appropriate policy options. Available data are often neither timely nor relevant, are provided long after they are needed, and do not address the problem. Sometimes there is also a dichotomy of need, interest, and perspective between the producer and user of the information. At the same time, the wide variety of analytic techniques available cause corollary problems. Some techniques need large quantities of data from multiple, diverse sources, while others are too complex to use easily. Moreover, too often the producer of information is enamored with the technique and does not focus on the results.

Substantial disagreement and confusion surround the usefulness of cost-benefit and cost-effectiveness analyses in decisions regarding medical technology introduction, use, and evaluation. Every medical technology has benefits, costs, and risks. The scientific answer is often equivocal; trade-offs must be made, and risks and costs estimated without the benefit of definitive results from large-scale investigations. Studies seldom provide a full picture of the efficacy, effectiveness, cost, risks, and benefits of a medical technology. Even so, decisions on use, and eventually on payment, must be made. All this takes place in intensely political environments.

To address these concerns, prescription drugs were chosen as the model medical technology because they offered the greatest analytic potential. The best available data on medical technology exist with prescription drugs because the Food and Drug Administration requires well-controlled studies that prove safety and efficacy before the product can be released for general marketing. Of all available drugs, cimetidine was chosen as the model not only because it met FDA requirements, but also because it recently underwent a range of well-designed cost-benefit and cost-effectiveness studies in many countries.

GOALS AND OBJECTIVES

The goal of the symposium was to present a generic effort of cost-benefit and cost-effectiveness analyses of medical technology that would aid policy planners and decision makers in their decision-making efforts. Six specific objectives were set:

1) Encourage a critical review of cost-benefit and cost-effectiveness analysis as a tool for policymaking.
2) Enhance utilization of timely and appropriate data and other research results useful in setting rational and effective policy.
3) Bring together researchers and health policymakers in a conference setting to exchange ideas and appreciate the efforts, needs, and requirements of others.
4) Identify cost-benefit and cost-effectiveness questions that are most important to those who set policy, particularly in the current environment of constrained resources.
5) Determine the best utilization of cost-benefit and cost-effectiveness analyses results as an aid in policymaking and policy implementation.
6) Increase communication and strengthen the informal network among researchers who undertake cost-benefit and cost-effectiveness studies, and the policymakers and providers who use or apply studies in helping to develop policies.

A diverse group of participants were invited from academic institutions, state and Federal governments, and nonprofit organizations from the United States and Europe. Policymakers and policy analysts comprised most of the group in order to allow the broadest possible spectrum of backgrounds, perspectives, and interests. This was also meant to encourage spirited interchange between the two main groups: information producers and information users. The assumption was that the results of this symposium would be especially helpful to decision makers in understanding and evaluating the usefulness, effects, and costs of medical technologies.

To encourage active participation by all attendees, the symposium was divided into two distinct, but closely related sections. First, four presentations were made during a plenary session. These dealt with the current status of research, policymaking problems at the Federal and state levels, and future directions for medical technology policymaking. After the presentations, all participants divided into nine concurrent groups convened to deal with issues raised by the presentations and to answer a set of specific questions developed by the Advisory Committee. The working group sessions were a significant element of the conference: it was hoped that the small (eight-member maximum) groups would be conducive to intense discussion and exchange.

Three sets of three working groups were arranged. Each small group was charged with reaching a consensus concerning one of the three specific policy areas. The three themes addressed were:

1) Use of cost-benefit and cost-effectiveness analysis in policymaking
2) Integration of research results with external factors in the policy and decision-making process
3) Priorities for future studies of medical technology

Each group had a facilitator whose responsibility was to formulate a group consensus. The three group facilitators, who were responsible for each theme, subsequently met to reach a consensus and present the synthesis at the final plenary session.

CHAPTER I

Overview and Summary

Bernard S. Bloom, Ph.D.

Background: CBA/CEA in Health Care

Presentations: Use and Acceptance of CBA/CEA, The Federal Political Environment, The State Political Environment, Future Uses of CBA/CEA

Summary of Working Group Sessions

Conference Summary

Overview and Summary

Bernard S. Bloom, Ph.D.

BACKGROUND

The use of cost-benefit and cost-effectiveness analyses (CBA/CEA) as an aid in policymaking has a long and generally beneficent history stretching back more than 3 centuries. During the third quarter of the 17th century, Sir William Petty suggested moving people out of London during the summer as an antidote to rampant illness.[1] Petty estimated that given the value of a human being plus the cost of transportation and care in the countryside for 3 months, every pound spent would yield a return of £84.

Nearly 2 centuries later in the United States, Lemuel Shattuck used a similar argument before the Massachusetts legislature for clean water and sanitary sewage disposal systems, required vaccination, and state and local boards of public health.[2] He argued that these deficiencies measurably reduced human productive capacity, thus robbing society of appreciable wealth. Shattuck estimated that 6,000 unnecessary deaths occurred each year in Massachusetts that could be attributed to public health deficiencies. Each death meant that an average of 18 years of productive life was unnecessarily lost at a value of $50 per year, or a total annual loss of $5.4 million. Additionally, he estimated 12,000 labor-years lost annually because of illness. Each year of lost productivity cost $100 plus $50 for treatment, or a total cost of $1.8 million. Finally, Shattuck estimated the cost of public support of widows and orphans at $1 per week for each worker who died, or a cost of $312,000. Thus, the total annual social cost was $7,512,000. Preventing these deaths by the recommended measures would yield, according to Shattuck's most conservative estimate, a return of $1,000 for every dollar spent.

Modern wide-scale use of CBA/CEA in the United States was introduced by the Army Corps of Engineers in their efforts to improve inland waterways. Its use became mandatory with the Flood Control Act of 1936, which required all projects begun under this Act to explicate costs and expected benefits before initiation.

CBA/CEA in Health Care

CBA/CEA in health care in the 20th century can be traced to a study by Dublin and Whitney, published in 1920.[3] They attributed cost to years of life lost because of tuberculosis and concluded that the loss of each year of life for all patients with tuberculosis represented a national economic loss of $26.5 billion. Additional losses not calculated were those due to morbidity, wages lost, and cost of medical and other care. The implicit assumption was that preventing and treating tuberculosis was highly cost effective.

CBA/CEA medical care studies are a recent phenomenon, less than 2 decades old. Some cost-effectiveness studies have dealt with surgical care (Piachaud and Weddell[4]; Velez-Gil et al[5]), coronary care units (Martin et al[6]; Bloom and Peterson[7]), and hypertension (Stason and Weinstein[8]). Cost-benefit studies have run the gamut from poliomyelitis vaccine (Weisbrod[9]) to estrogen use in postmenopausal women (Weinstein[10]). Although the main thrust of these studies has been to influence policy at a micro level (physician decisions regarding a specific disease or therapy or an individual patient or practice), there are also macro-policy implications (that which is deemed beneficial for one patient is often the appropriate policy [care] for all similar patients).

PRESENTATIONS

Use and Acceptance of CBA/CEA

The most recent emphasis of CBA/CEA has been to influence policy and policymakers directly. The assumption in rational policymaking is that good information can affect policy option development and decisions. For this to succeed, the three key decision makers in the medical care interchange, ie, providers, consumers, and third-party payers, must be willing to accept and use CBA/CEA results. Dr. Duncan Neuhauser considers this to be the first and most important prerequisite. At the least, these key decision makers must feel confident with study results, which in turn must reflect data obtained by well-controlled studies determining efficacy and effectiveness. They must also include an awareness of cost side effects. For instance, if side effects exceed benefits for some patients, they may withdraw from treatment, thus reducing total benefits.

Recognizing the difference between efficacy and effectiveness is also of paramount importance and highlights the differences between results in the experimental world (efficacy) and real world (effectiveness). CBA/CEA require comparisons not only with placebo or no treatment (the experimental world) but with the next best alternative (the real world).

There is little question that cimetidine is an excellent model to illustrate the successful application of CBA/CEA. It is one of the best evaluated medical technologies and meets acceptance by the three key decision makers. The major concern is whether other medical interventions will pass such exhaustive investigation. Only rarely will a case argue so strongly in favor of using CBA/CEA in policymaking. This might not be of such major concern if our experience were greater with the full range of intense investigation early in the medical technology life-cycle. Cimetidine is the first to be studied in this way, but hopefully the first of many.

The Federal Political Environment

The history of U.S. government involvement in medical technology evaluation can best be described as sporadic. In response to a highly publicized problem, a period of intense interest is followed by one of decreased emphasis. The growing usefulness and acceptance of CBA/CEA as a health care policymaking tool, especially among academicians and researchers, raises a question as to whether government policy analysts and policymakers are prepared to utilize these techniques for medical technology decision making in their respective political environments. The Congressional Office of Technology Assessment (OTA) concluded that at their present state of development, CBA/CEA are best used as adjuncts to decision making rather than as policy determinants.

This evaluation ebb and flow began at the turn of the 20th century with Federal government concern over adulterated foods and mislabeling of pharmaceutical preparations, as Dr. Joyce Lashof described in her presentation. The Federal role has changed over time as medical technology innovation has increased and become more complex. Recently, the major emphasis has been on the responsibility of the Food and Drug Administration in guaranteeing product safety and efficacy. A new thrust appears to be developing wherein cost-effectiveness analysis is being relied on more frequently by OTA in its analysis of medical care problems and development of policy options.

As more Federal agencies address economic, social, and ethical issues, in addition to problems of safety and efficacy, there arises a lack of clear roles and responsibilities in medical technology evaluation. Interest in using CBA/CEA in both assessment and policy option development is currently increasing in a number of agencies. However, this does not suggest that CBA/CEA are universally accepted or utilized. In fact, there are no requirements for their use, and they are considered by some a burdensome addition to the regulatory requirements in the approval of drugs and medical devices.

The State Political Environment

Along with the results of CBA/CEA, policymakers must be aware of the political environment wherein decisions are to be made. Frequently, Congress places paramount emphasis on political considerations, overriding scientific medical technology assessment. In effect, Congress uses its own informal methods of CBA/CEA for policy-making.

The conflicting relation between scientific results of CBA/CEA and political exigencies cannot be stressed too strongly. As Myrle Myers so cogently argued, marked differences exist between public and private sector decision making. The private sector is geared to maximizing profit, while the prime concern of the public sector is minimizing programmatic costs.

The policy decision-making process regarding medical technology usage and payment at the state level often contains certain informal features of CBA/CEA. Although it is often recognized that formal CBA/CEA can be used to determine the value and usefulness of a specific program, decisions are rarely based on these analyses. However, the political climate may be changing as radically as the economic one. And, since demand will continue to exceed supply in the immediate future, the probability increases that CBA/CEA may play a larger political role in the current constrained budget atmosphere. Nevertheless, this does not mean that these decisions will be based entirely on CBA/CEA. Moreover, moral and emotional issues add to the political and economic concerns in public policy decision making. The constant struggle in the political arena detracts from the ability to use CBA/CEA and other research results in determining policy. Results from CBA/CEA that emphasize areas or programs at less cost may be more favorably received in an era of tight budgets.

Future Uses of CBA/CEA

Heretofore, research results have been aimed at administrators, policy analysts, and policymakers. Not only must CBA/CEA deal with both issues and problems important to policymakers, but future results must be aimed beyond the traditional policymakers to include other constituencies, ie, the general public, politicians, and other interest groups.

Changing governmental priorities, programs, and funding as well as slowed economic growth provide an opportunity for expanding the role of CBA/CEA in policymaking. As Dr. Paul Stolley noted, the need for good studies will be more important than ever. The basis of CBA/CEA must still be grounded in well-controlled investigations of efficacy, without which it will be impossible to provide good estimates of medical care effects or benefits.

Despite efforts at improving results, CBA/CEA will still remain less than the perfect policymaking tool. The precise evaluation of costs and effects, especially many of the indirect costs, benefits, and risks, will continue to be difficult. Methods of calculating costs, risks, benefits, and side effects will be subject to differences of opinion. Interpretation of results will remain another contentious issue; and difficulties in identifying and evaluating major policy effects will continue to arise. However, these difficulties need not deter us from continuing to expand CBA/CEA use and usefulness.

Dr. Stolley also noted a few caveats and suggestions for future CBA/CEA use. First, reliance should be increased on nontraditional methods of obtaining data and research results to supplement and complement randomized controlled clinical trials of safety and efficacy, eg, increased use of case-control studies, cohort studies, quasi-experimental designs, and postmarketing surveillance. Second, cost-effectiveness analyses of health programs should precede cost-benefit analyses. With the good methodologies currently available for determining direct cost, benefits, effects, and risks, emphasis should turn to the intangibles and indirect costs and effects in these areas. Furthermore, Dr. Stolley stressed the need to implement only medical technologies that have been adequately and appropriately evaluated and are of known benefit.

SUMMARY OF WORKING GROUP SESSIONS

Symposium participants chose one of nine small working groups, each led by a facilitator, and were charged to answer predetermined questions developed by the National Advisory Committee. Each set of questions was built around one of the three major symposium themes. After the working groups had completed their task, the three facilitators responsible for each theme met to reach further consensus. They elected a representative to present the theme consensus in the final plenary session. The key points agreed upon in the working group sessions presented are summarized below by theme.

Theme I:
Use of CBA/CEA in Policymaking— Harvey V. Fineberg, M.D., Ph.D.

1) CBA/CEA should emphasize the societal perspective, although it was recognized that many other perspectives need to be considered. These include executive and legislative branches of government, patients and other consumers, providers, third-party payers, and industrial payers of insurance premiums.
2) All costs and benefits need to be accounted for, no matter who is affected.
3) A range of disciplines must be included in the analyses, eg, economics, statistics, epidemiology, and medicine.
4) Priority should be given to current, practical policymaking needs in order for CBA/CEA to deal with pressing problems.
5) The varied individual and group perspectives and values have to be considered in any consensus regarding CBA/CEA results.
6) An additional objective of CBA/CEA might be to reinforce societal values.
7) Methodologic limitations of CBA/CEA are related to timeliness of results, divergence of decision-maker and analyst perspectives, changing

political environments, lack of appropriate data bearing on specific problems, and emphasis on evaluation of new medical technology at the expense of existing technology.

8) Vested interests were recognized as an additional barrier to utilizing the results of CBA/CEA.

9) Objectivity of CBA/CEA and credibility of research are the best assurance of acceptance by policymakers.

10) Occasionally, rapid but incomplete analyses leading to a conclusion can be useful.

11) Policy decision makers need training in CBA/CEA to understand its uses and limitations in order to implement results more effectively.

12) Conversely, policy analysts and researchers should be aware of the needs and perspectives of decision makers.

13) Valuable lessons were obtained from the cimetidine model:

    a) Importance of combining clinical trials and epidemiological studies along with CBA/CEA in evaluating any new medical technology.

    b) Importance of identifying alternatives when weighing costs, benefits, and effects of a particular medical technology.

    c) Importance of understanding changes in the evolution or natural history of the underlying disease process.

    d) Recognizing "technology creep," a medical technology designed for specific uses that is soon utilized in other marginally beneficial areas.

    e) Recognizing that cimetidine is an unusual example of a medical technology because its cost and risk are reduced at the same time; everyone (providers, consumers, and payers) profits from these circumstances.

Theme II:
Integration of Research Results With External Factors in the Policy- and Decision-Making Process—
James T. Doluisio, Ph.D.

1) Three basic and distinct policy decision-making models utilize CBA/CEA:

    a) Decisions made by executive and legislative branches through the appropriations process and primarily affecting Medicaid.

    b) Decisions made by the Food and Drug Administration through the approval process affecting those who market and those who utilize drugs and medications.

    c) Specification of the general models and the information needed by various groups for policy decision making.

2) The credibility of researchers and data is of prime importance in acceptance and use of CBA/CEA by policymakers.

3) Since the future guarantees more complex decision-making problems, previous informal decision-making processes cannot solely be relied on.

4) A basic requirement of decision makers is timely data that include both direct and indirect effects.

5) CBA/CEA will be relied on more frequently if state and Federal budgetary constraints plus slowed economic growth continue as expected.

6) Although CBA/CEA was recognized as a potentially useful aid in policymaking, their own effectiveness has not been proven to everyone's satisfaction.

7) CBA/CEA can be used in rational policymaking by influencing politicians and other public decision makers, as well as in dealing with special or vested interest groups.

Theme III:
Priorities for Future Studies of Medical Technology—
Clifton A. Cole, M.P.A.

1) CBA/CEA are only two of a number of techniques useful to evaluate medical technology.

2) A weakness of CBA/CEA is reliance on retrospective data.

3) Future models should be automated so that CBA/CEA can be undertaken simultaneously with other evaluation studies using prospective data.

4) Current data on CBA/CEA are insufficient for many medical technologies and medical interventions.

5) Even with inherent weaknesses, CBA/CEA should be used more frequently than at present by policymakers.

6) Additional studies testing costs, benefits, and effects of medical technology can be extended to other conditions for which that technology may be used.

7) Long-term follow-up studies are needed to confirm initial results in order to uncover differences between efficacy and effectiveness.

8) Postmarketing surveillance is important, primarily to detect previously unknown or unsuspected costs, risks, and benefits.

9) Closer cooperation between private sector and government research efforts, while recognizing differing needs and perspectives, would be less costly and mutually beneficial.

10) Greater cooperation is needed between state and Federal governments and among agencies within each level for more efficient and effective research resource allocation, sharing of knowledge, and joint public policymaking.

11) CBA/CEA will ultimately be evaluated by its effects on decision making. If these tools aid decision makers, they will be seen as useful and reliable.

CONFERENCE SUMMARY

Synthesizing or summarizing the products of nine working groups, which comprised about 70 people working intensively over 2 days, is a particularly difficult task. I visited nearly all the working groups at least once. I also heard each facilitator present a synthesis of his theme consensus. At least nine basic issues could be identified. These are the common threads running through the output of all working group sessions.

The first one is that we have all recognized the problems of resource allocation and that all resources ultimately are finite; that we are faced with immediate and severe resource restrictions in health and medical care services and are aware of the effects of budgetary constraints on the populations served. The emphasis now is on cost control at all government levels. In the past we have relied on intuitive decision-making processes to arrive at what we thought were the best possible policy decisions. However, the future requires more quantitative approaches to setting more rational policies, and more efficient and effective ways of distributing our increasingly constrained resource base.

The second theme concluded that there is general acceptance of cost-benefit and cost-effectiveness analyses as being helpful in making policy decisions and in understanding their first and second order effects. However, a cautionary note was injected time and again: that we should not have unrealistic expectations of CBA or CEA. It is only one of many tools that decision makers can use. It neither makes decisions nor does it relieve policymakers of the responsibilities for making decisions. We must continue to rely on the sound judgment and wisdom of public decision makers.

The third theme showed that although CBA and CEA have rather variable effects on decision making, they may be more or less successful in helping decision makers. There was a high level of awareness in recognizing that political concerns often overwhelm any attempts at rational public decision making. The well-documented results from CBA/CEA or any other good study may be ignored in the cauldron of conflicting interests known as the political arena.

The fourth, which surprised me, although in retrospect it should not have, was that CBA/CEA are usually viewed as a whole, or two sides of the same coin, even though it was recognized that there are definitional and methodological differences.

The fifth theme stressed that CBA and CEA results, like any study results, must be timely, understandable, useful, and usable to decision makers. Academicians and researchers must, either in concert with decision makers or through effective use of the crystal ball, be able to predict when appropriate studies should be undertaken so that information can be available to decision makers. As a corollary, the results of any studies should be widely distributed beyond that at present in academic or other narrowly focused journals.

The sixth theme emphasized the need for a wedding of interests, expertise, and understanding of both academicians and researchers on the one hand and policymakers on the other; that CBA/CEA, like all studies, should be designed and carried out by teams made up of members from both groups. The existing arrangement that researchers develop and execute studies and then give the information to the decision makers is no longer the best method. Rather, there should be a team approach to these studies, with both groups having input at all stages of design, implementation, and analyses.

The seventh theme was that CBA/CEA seem to be embraced more enthusiastically by academicians and researchers than policymakers for what is believed to be their prima facie value. This should not be considered unusual. In other areas where cost-benefit and cost-effectiveness analyses have been used for longer periods of time, such as in defense or flood control and other water projects, it took many years for these studies to be accepted and utilized. We in academia should not feel particularly uncomfortable. CBA/CEA have only been used in health care for less than 20 years. Perhaps it will take a generation for broad acceptance and utilization.

The eighth theme was that CBA/CEA alone should not be expected to solve problems. They are not the only research tool; other studies, for example, case control or cohort studies and other postmarketing surveillance techniques, are useful as well. These complement CBA/CEA and the randomized controlled trials of efficacy and effectiveness. The major emphasis of all studies undertaken to assist decision makers should be on outcome or output. Process evaluations have an important place, but they should not predominate.

The last theme stressed that although programmatic approaches may be useful to individual decision makers, we should neither lose sight of the wider application of study results nor neglect effects of decisions on the wider society, and on the social, political, and economic milieu within which all decisions are ultimately made.

REFERENCES

1. Hull CH (ed): *The Economic Writings of Sir William Petty.* Cambridge, England, Cambridge University Press, 1899
2. Shattuck L: *Report of the Sanitary Commission of Massachusetts. 1850.* Cambridge, Mass, Harvard University Press, 1948
3. Dublin LI, Whitney J: The costs of tuberculosis. *Publications of the American Statistical Association* 17:441–450, 1920
4. Piachaud D, Weddell JM: Cost of treating varicose veins. *Lancet* 2:1191–1192, 1972
5. Velez-Gil A et al: A simplified system for surgical operations: The economics of treating hernia. *Surgery* 77:391–394, 1975
6. Martin SP et al: Inputs into coronary care during 30 years: A cost effectiveness study. *Annals of Internal Medicine* 81:289–293, 1974
7. Bloom BS, Peterson OL: End results, cost and productivity of coronary care units. *New England Journal of Medicine* 302:938–942, 1973
8. Stason WB, Weinstein M: Allocation of resources to manage hypertension. *New England Journal of Medicine* 296:732–739, 1977
9. Weisbrod BA: Costs and benefits of medical research: A case study of poliomyelitis. *Journal of Political Economy* 79:527–544, 1971
10. Weinstein M: Estrogen use in postmenopausal women: Costs, risk and benefits. *New England Journal of Medicine* 303:308–316, 1980

CHAPTER II

Invited Presentations

Survey of Research Results and Current Status of CBA/CEA in Technology Assessment: Cimetidine as a Model
Duncan Neuhauser, Ph.D.

Discussion

Medical Technology Decision Making in a Political Environment at the Federal Level
Joyce C. Lashof, M.D.

Discussion

Medical Technology Decision Making in a Political Environment at the State Level
Myrle A. Myers, R.Ph., M.S.

Discussion

Priorities for Future CBA/CEA in Policymaking
Paul D. Stolley, M.D.

Discussion

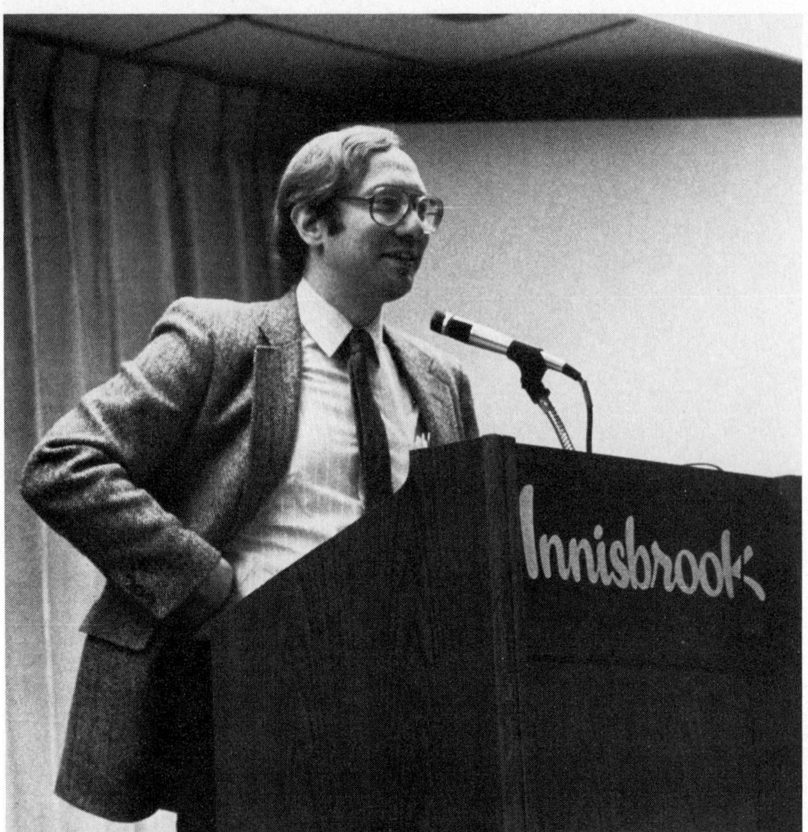

Harvey Fineberg, M.D. Ph.D.

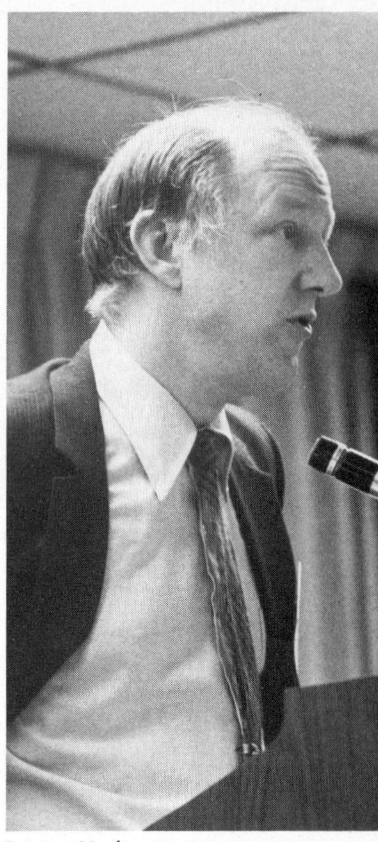

Duncan Neuhauser, Ph.D.

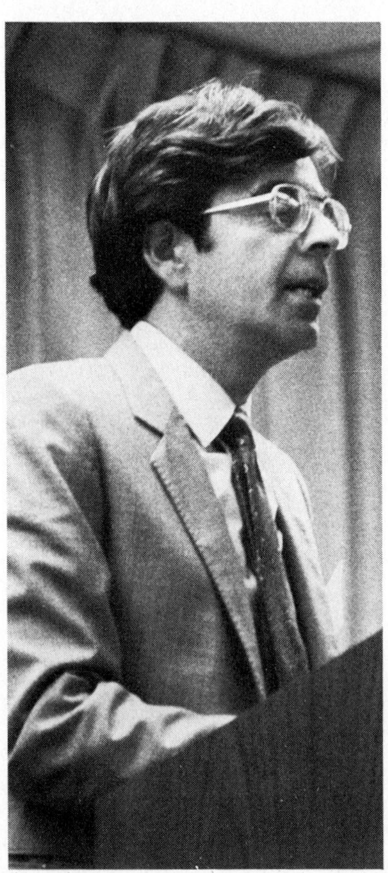

Bernard S. Bloom, Ph.D.

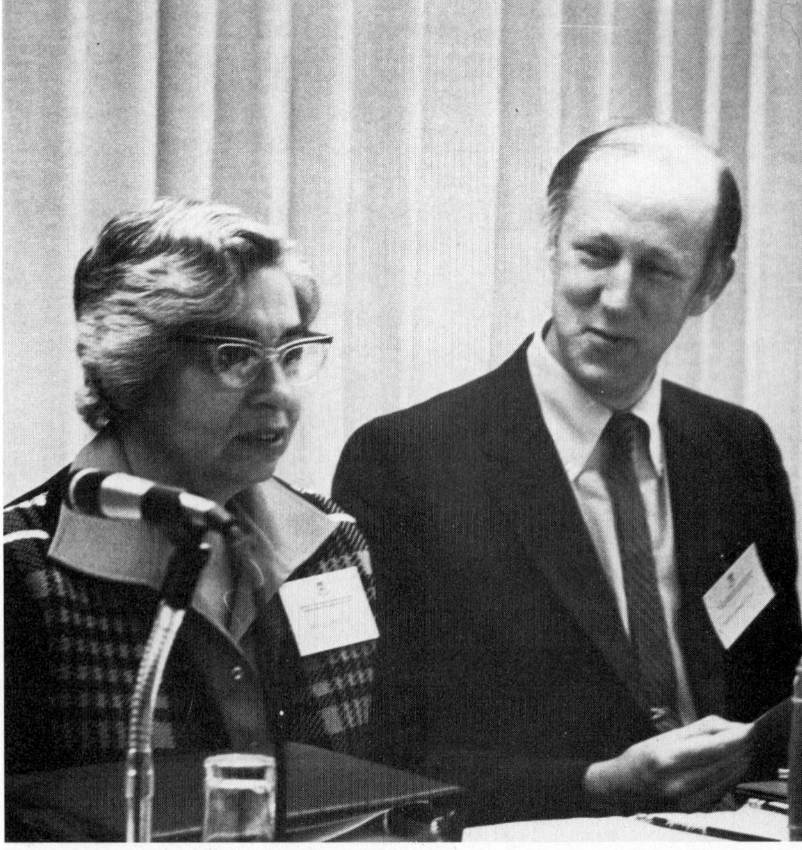

Joyce C. Lashof, M.D; Duncan Neuhauser, Ph.D.

Photos: Janis R. Nollendorfs

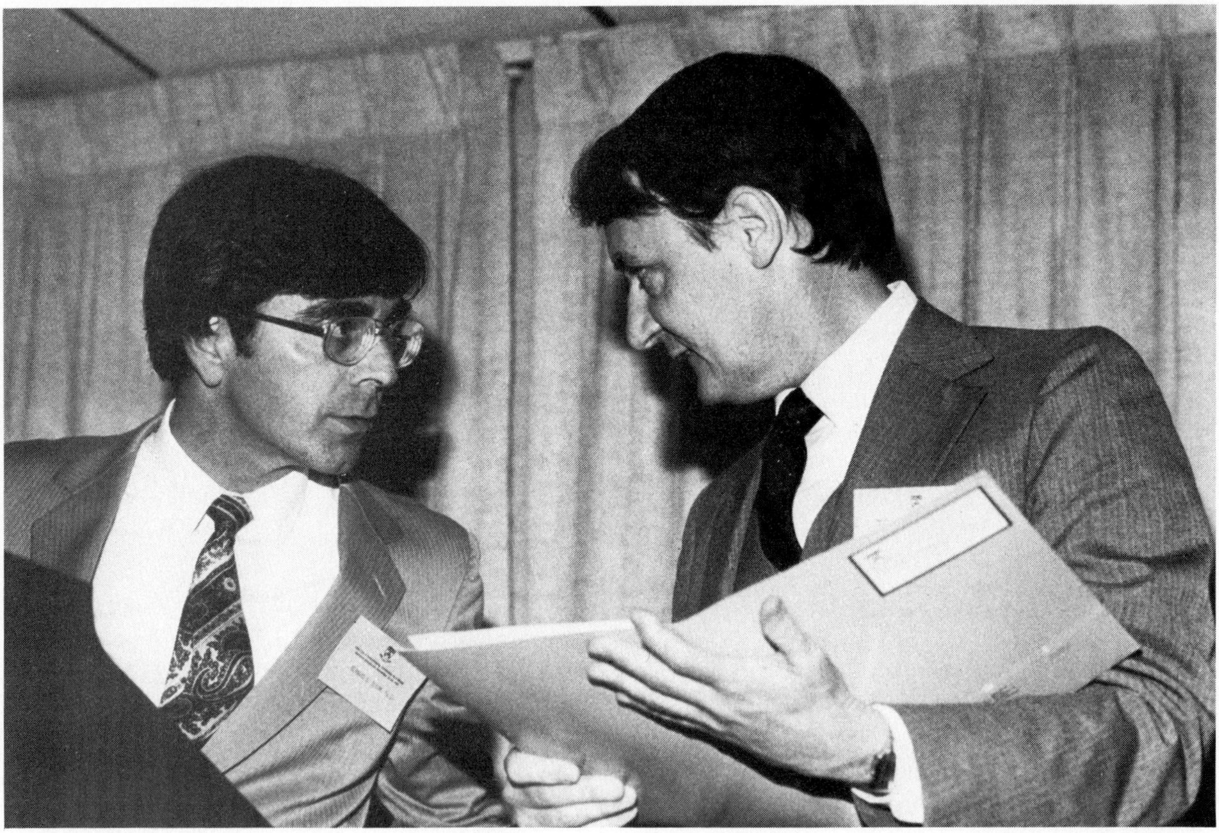

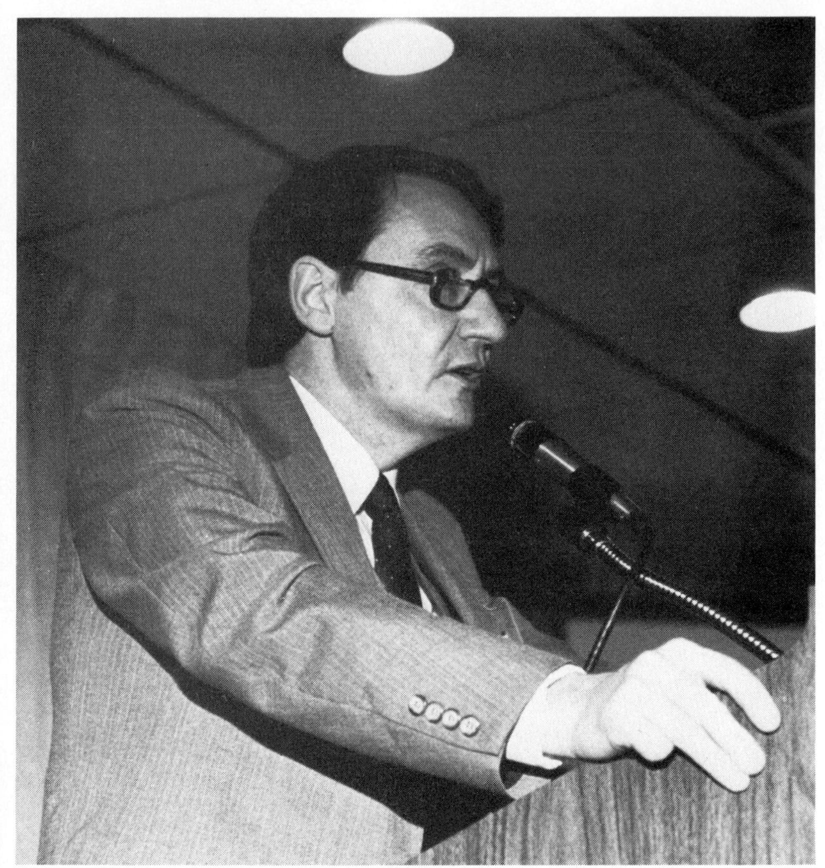

(l-r) Bernard S. Bloom, Ph.D.; William P. Pierskalla, Ph.D.

William P. Pierskalla, Ph.D.

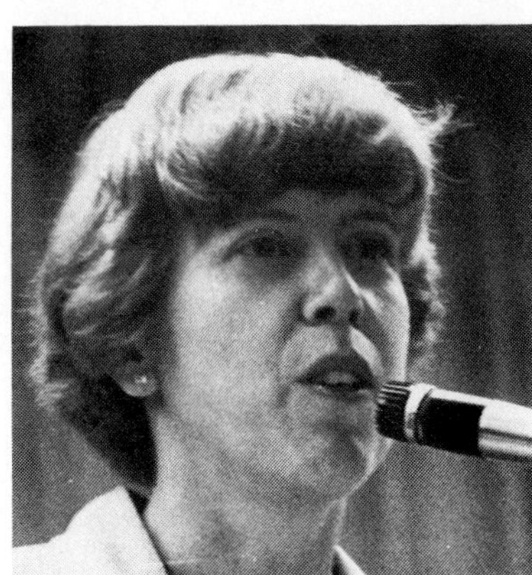

Myrle A. Myers, R.Ph.

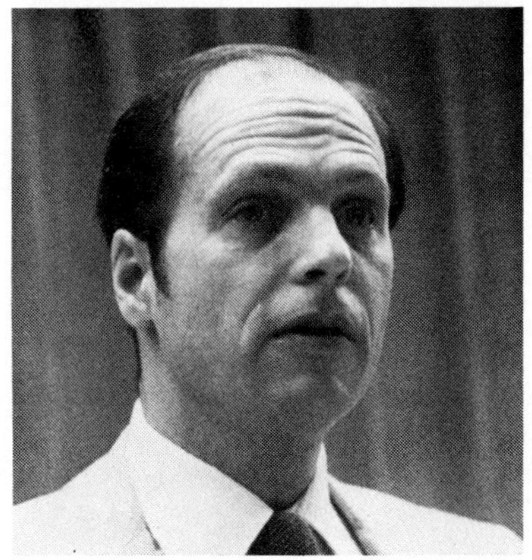

Paul D. Stolley, M.D.

Survey of Research Results and Current Status of CBA/CEA in Technology Assessment: Cimetidine as a Model

Duncan Neuhauser, Ph.D.

Professor of Epidemiology and Community Health
Professor of Medicine, Case Western Reserve University
Cleveland, Ohio

INTRODUCTION

Stated simply, cimetidine is a good thing. The questions at hand are: How sure are we that this is true? How much of a good thing? For whom? And finally at a different level of analysis, can the evaluation of cimetidine be applied usefully to other medical interventions?

Cimetidine as a Model

Perhaps more effort has gone into analyzing the costs and benefits of cimetidine than any other medical intervention. Could such efforts usefully be applied to other medical interventions? Once the Food and Drug Administration (FDA) has approved a drug, several additional decision makers are required in order for the drug to be accepted. Third party payers, providers, and patients, must each be willing to use the medical intervention in question. Cimetidine may reduce third party costs (+), is a treatment providers believe to be efficacious (+), and a treatment patients accept (+). These desirable attributes generally do not exist for other medical interventions. Coronary artery bypass graft is accepted by surgeons (+) and patients (+) but has probably raised costs for third party payers (−). Regular dental flossing would probably lower third party costs (+), is advocated by dentists (+), but is not widely accepted by patients (−). It is important to remember these three decision-making groups when assessing the value of cost-benefit and cost-effectiveness analyses of medical interventions.

How Sure Are We?

Answering this question requires a review of the scientific literature, specifically the clinical trials in which cimetidine was given to some patients and not others. The trick is to design a trial ensuring that all possible effects on outcome are eliminated, with the exception of cimetidine. Two similar trials are better than one. However, questions arise about how to compare them, particularly if they produce different results (Figure 1).

Key Components of a Clinical Trial

Although randomization of patients into experimental and control groups is the best method, similarity of the groups is not a certainty. A clear definition of the type of patient being treated is also useful. The term double-blind implies that both the patient and the physician are unaware of whether they are getting or giving the experimental therapy, standard therapy or just a placebo, an inert agent with no chemical effect on the disease. After some lapse of time the patient's disease is evaluated, ideally by a physician who does not know whether the patient is in the control (placebo) or experimental groups. This design reduces the possibility of physician or patient bias for or against the treatment. The physician's bias has little room to operate if the end state is "alive" or "dead," but it may be important if the outcome evaluation measures relief of pain, patient anxiety, or satisfaction with care. Evaluating the adequacy of trials is a subjective process open to different interpretation and based in part on the medical specialist's prior expectations.

THE CIMETIDINE-DUODENAL ULCER TRIALS

The Hibbard and Strom literature review[1] reported 22 placebo-controlled studies for short-term therapy of cimetidine for duodenal ulcer, of which

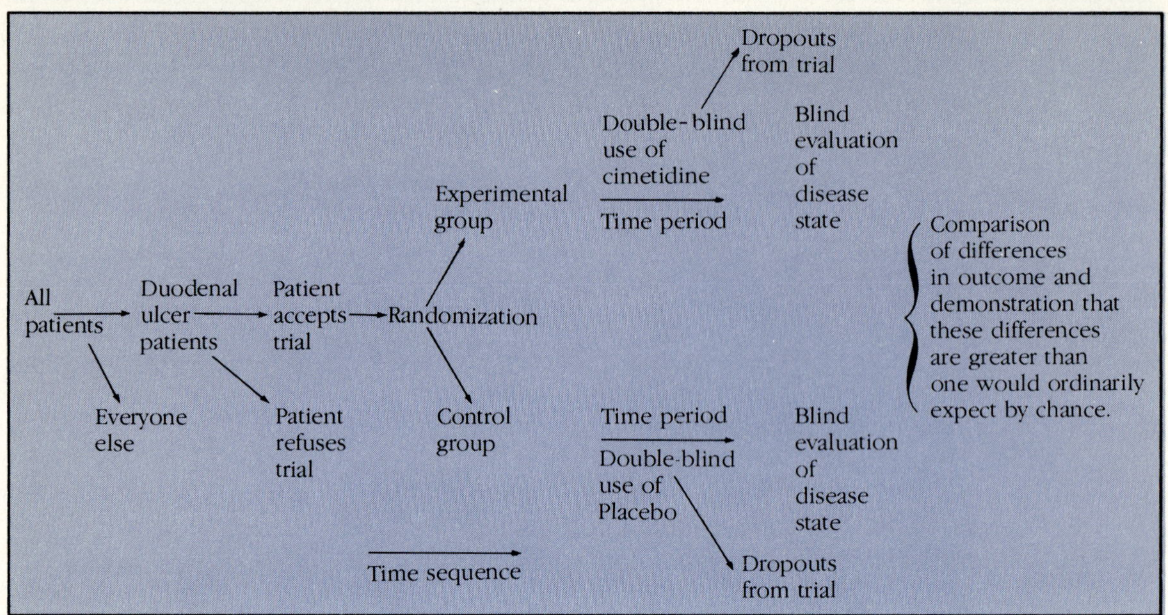

Figure 1. Flow diagram of key components of double-blind randomized clinical trial for cimetidine and duodenal ulcer.

16 were randomized and 15 were both randomized and double-blind. Therapy lasted from 3 to 6 weeks.[2-23] Each study showed improvement with cimetidine compared with the placebo. Sixteen studies showed statistically significant differences in favor of cimetidine (4 of 15 randomized double-blind trials were not significant while 11 were significant). The Hibbard and Strom review reported another 12 placebo-controlled trials for long-term therapy, 10 of which were both randomized and double-blind.[24-35] Therapy lasted from 3 to 12 months. Each of the 12 studies showed improved results with cimetidine. Nine were significant at the 0.01 level.

The volume of consistent studies noted above makes cimetidine one of the best clinically evaluated medical interventions. Additionally, some variation in design adds to our belief in efficacy. Dosage levels varied from 0.8 to 1.6 g per day for the short-term studies and from 0.4 to 0.8 g per day for long-term studies. Evaluation for duodenal ulcer was by endoscopic assessment. In no study did the experimental group exceed 100 patients. Thus, treatment differences had to be large in order to demonstrate persistent, significant differences.

Follow-up periods. Follow-up was relatively short because an early effect was achieved. Bodemar and Walan[36] reported a trial from Linköping, Sweden with the longest follow-up period of 2 years. Twenty-two of 35 placebo patients participating in the study required operation at 2 years as compared with only 3 of 31 in the cimetidine group.

It should be noted that some interventions require long time periods to understand their range of impact. The risks of x-ray exposure, for example, were known 20 years after the discovery of the x-ray itself. Control of these risks took 40 years, and we are still debating the effects of small exposure levels 85 years later.

The placebo effect. These studies compare cimetidine with a placebo. The placebo effect was large, with roughly 40% of patients "cured" compared with approximately 80% of the cimetidine patients. The placebo effect can be achieved by at least six phenomena[37,38]: (1) the impact of patient belief on physiological functioning, (2) the patient's perception of symptoms, (3) the patient's desire to please the physician by over-reporting positive results, (4) the examining physician's optimistic bias in reporting improvement, (5) the patient's spontaneous recovery, called "regression to the mean," and (6) other traditional treatments (antacid use) or behavior change (diet change) that influence recovery. These effects seem to cure 40% of duodenal ulcer patients.

Side effects or risks. In the trials, 1.5% of patients receiving cimetidine required withdrawal of treatment, compared with 1.2% of those receiving placebo. Seventeen percent of cimetidine patients reported untoward signs and symptoms not requiring withdrawal compared to 19% of

18

placebo patients. These side effects would appear to be reversible, and this reversibility is important for cost-benefit and cost-effectiveness analyses. If side effects exceed the benefits for some patients, then these patients may withdraw from treatment, thus reducing the percent of patients benefiting.

Withdrawal from treatment. Side effects are only one reason for withdrawal from treatment. Failure to comply and increased severity of disease compelling other treatment, in this case surgical operation, are additional reasons for withdrawal from treatment.

Any operation while correcting the disease has mortality, side effects, pain, and high costs. For these reasons it should be considered a negative outcome in the trials.

CIMETIDINE AND THE ALTERNATIVES

Twenty-two trials compared cimetidine to placebo, to the former's advantage (Figure 2). The placebo comparison tests the benefit that exceeds a psychological threshold. That is, the drug must exceed the placebo driven power of imagination. This exacting standard may not be appropriate for cost-benefit analysis. Cost-benefit analysis requires comparing it with the next best alternative, which would otherwise have been used. Two existing alternatives to cimetidine are antacids and surgical operation. Three trials comparing antacids and cimetidine failed to demonstrate a statistically significant difference in benefit. Two somewhat different trials compared antacids with placebo: one showed no significant difference; the other showed a significant difference in favor of antacids. (A new treatment, colloidal bismuth, may be as efficacious as cimetidine. However, it has yet to be evaluated in humans.[39]) An operation is not a first treatment and is only used after failure of drug therapy. Therefore, a direct comparison would be inappropriate. However, comparing the benefits of surgical intervention with failure of drug therapy is a relevant clinical question.

While operation is a possibility, it is less likely for cimetidine users than for patients using its competing alternatives. When considering the effects of treatment, one must use some single scale to aggregate the different outcome states shown to the right of the branch points in Figure 3. In theory this can be achieved by utility analysis. For cost-benefit analysis, a monetary yardstick must be used. The cimetidine and traditional therapy choices in the decision tree in Figure 3 have a similar structure, but the branches have different probabilities (percentages) of occurrence.

The percentages shown come from a 1980 review by Piper.[44] Cimetidine compared with placebo may reduce the need for operation between threefold and sixfold and perhaps more. The trials, by their design, were carefully controlled. The real use of cimetidine may be quite different and this is important to keep in mind when moving to the cost-benefit and cost-effectiveness analyses that try to measure effects in the uncontrolled "real world."

COST-BENEFIT AND COST-EFFECTIVE-NESS ANALYSES

A cost-effectiveness analysis relates the dollar costs of care to a unit of outcome not measured in dollars, such as years of life saved, or days lost from work. A cost-benefit analysis compares the dollar costs of care with the outcome (benefit) measured in dollars. Its advantage is that it shows the net dollar savings, but it requires a subjective transformation of outcomes like quantity and quality of life into an acceptable dollar value.

One of the fundamental peculiarities of medical care is the effect of health insurance on patients, providers, insurers, and society's decision making. Health insurance releases the patient from financial responsibility for some care. A patient may pay more for outpatient cimetidine care than inpatient surgical procedure. The third party insurer does not directly need to take into account the change in productivity of workers as a result of eliminating a disease. Productivity is important for the society as a whole. It is customary that a cost-benefit analysis be carried out from a social perspective. This has been done for cimetidine.

However, the cost-benefit comparison is different than for the trials. The cost-benefit analyses have compared costs and benefits before and after the introduction of cimetidine (August 1977, in the United States), to decide its effects. Such a comparison assumes that nothing else has changed; this will be considered later. Furthermore, there is often a time lag between care expenditures and benefit realization, ie, some treatments might allow patients to die later in more expensive ways. Discounting is the usual method of relating present and future costs and benefits.

Defining the Patient Population

There are two types of peptic ulcer: duodenal and gastric (stomal ulcers are rare enough to be set aside). Duodenal ulcers approximate 80% of peptic ulcers, consume 70% of the medical care costs, and account for half the deaths (Table 1).

Some of the cost-benefit studies focused on the peptic ulcer population, which includes both

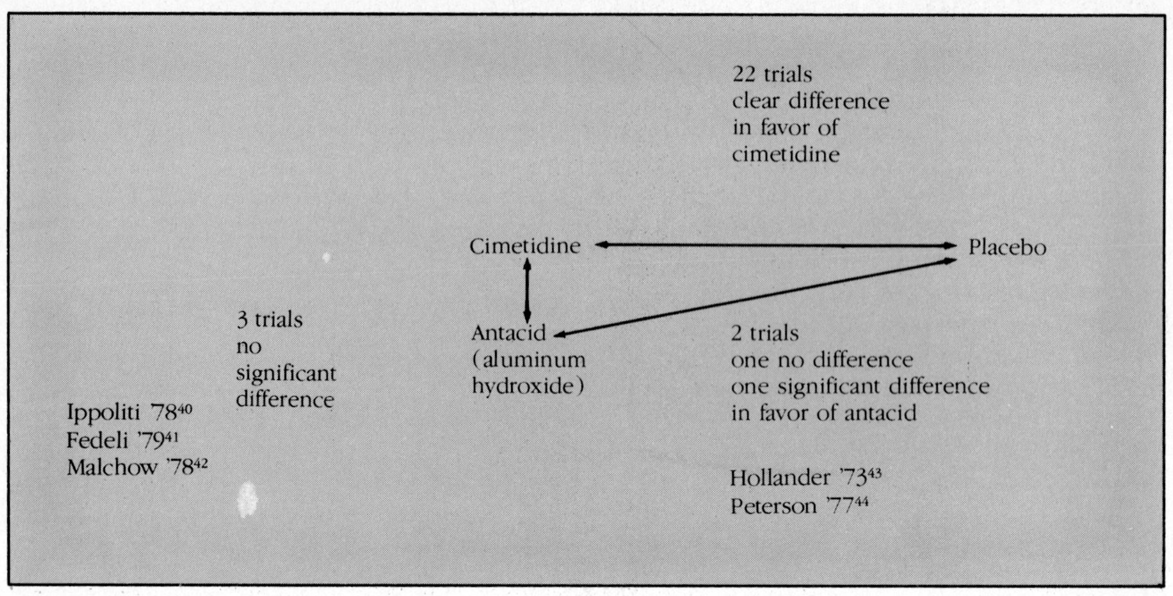

Figure 2. The comparison of three possible therapies for duodenal ulcer.

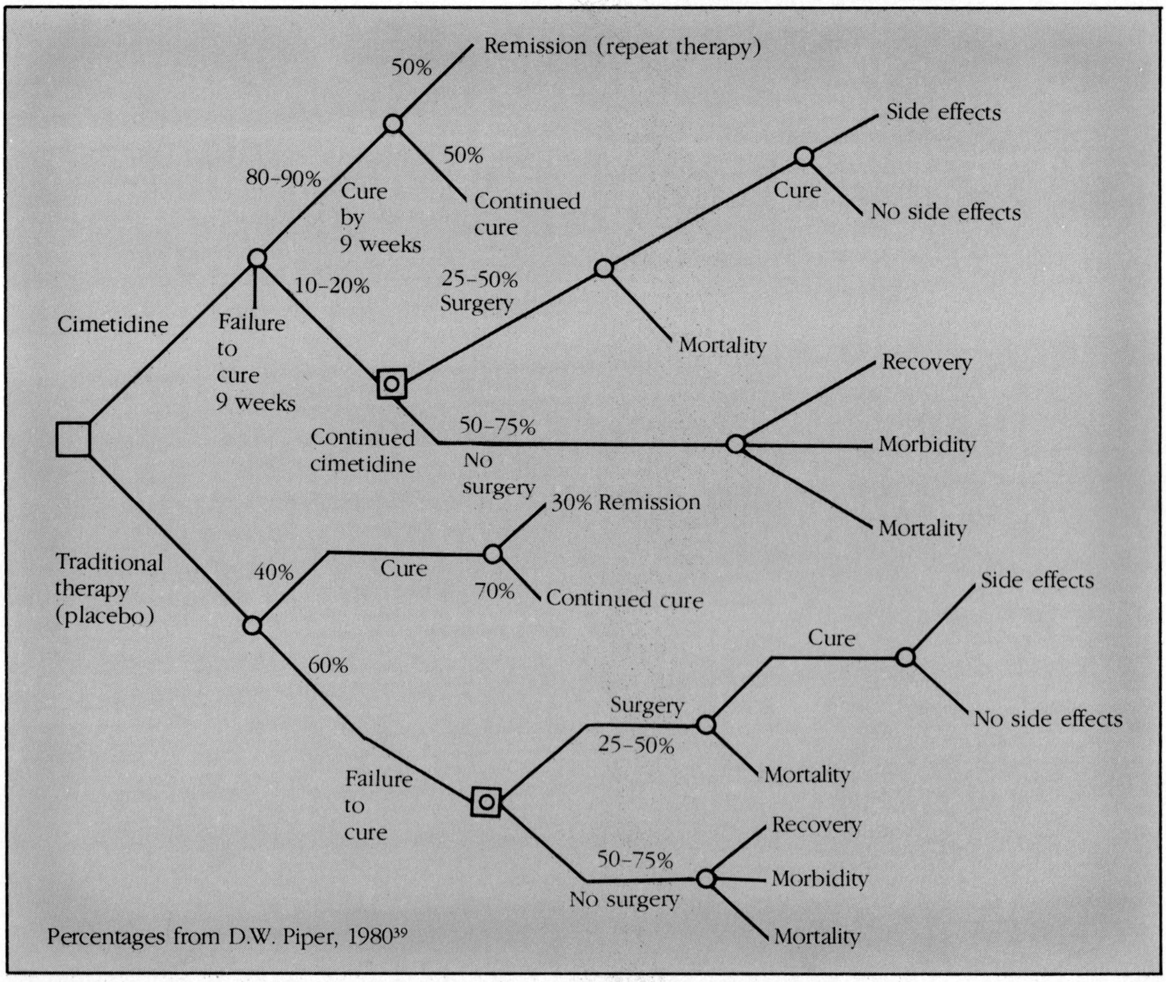

Figure 3. Comparing the effects of cimetidine and traditional therapy (placebo).

gastric and duodenal ulcers. The clinical trials reviewed so far have studied only those with duodenal ulcer. The FDA has approved cimetidine for use only on duodenal ulcers and Zollinger-Ellison syndrome. Fineberg and Pearlman[46] reviewed four short-term, double-blind placebo-controlled clinical trials on cimetidine and gastric ulcers.[47-50] All showed results favoring cimetidine, but only two were statistically significant. Piper, in summarizing cimetidine's effects, stated that it "is probably less dramatic in the case of chronic gastric ulcer than chronic duodenal ulcer."[39]

This use of cimetidine on other types of ulcers is important to remember with regard to the cost-benefit studies and may or may not be appropriate. There is inadequate evidence to judge.

Strategies for Treatment of Gastric Pain

The patient presents to the physician with pain and other ulcer symptoms. The physician may first diagnose and then treat. If unsuccessful, the physician will again diagnose or wait and see if the symptoms remain or get worse. He may then diagnose and treat or treat and diagnose.

These strategies are outlined in the decision tree shown in Figure 4. This tree must be viewed as approximate. The publication of Dr. Leighton Reads' more definitive study is awaited. The wait-

Table 1

Types Of Peptic Ulcers, Frequency and Costs[45]

	Frequency	Costs of care	Ulcer deaths 1975
Duodenal ulcer	80%	70%	50%
Gastric ulcer	20%	30%	50%
Total	100%	100%	100%

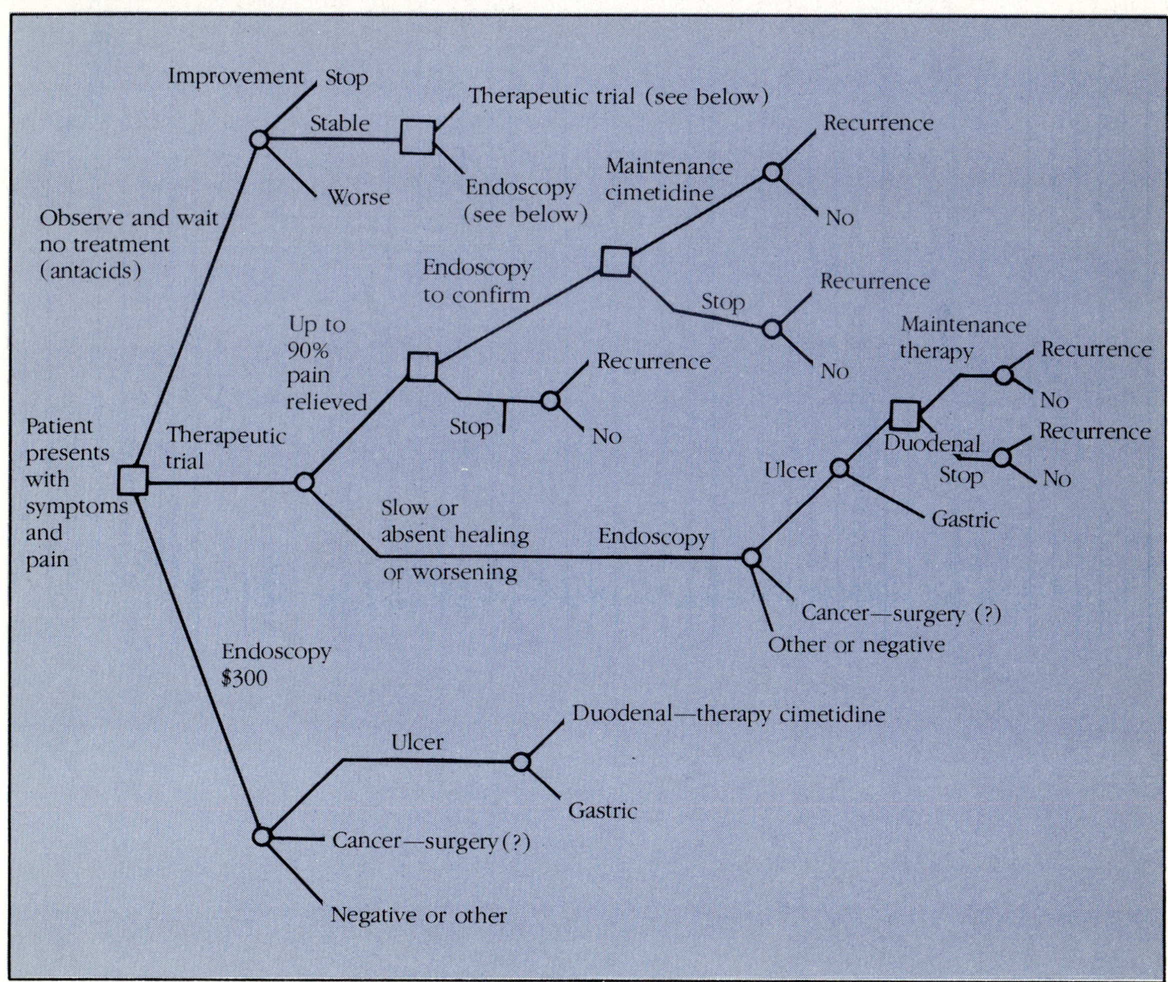

Figure 4. Decision tree for three alternative strategies for patients with gastric pain.

and-see strategy may be most appropriate when symptoms are minimal. There are two diagnostic tests—endoscopy (costs $200 to $300) and barium x-rays (upper GI series, costs $150). The latter are less accurate. It may be cost-effective to treat with cimetidine without testing (a "therapeutic trial"). If pain and symptoms are slow to heal or fail to heal, then endoscopy can be used to distinguish between gastric and duodenal ulcers, cancer, other, or no detectable disease. If this therapy-first strategy is applied, gastric ulcer patients, and even patients without ulcer disease, would be treated this way. Thus, it may be cost-effective to treat all patients with other diseases before testing. Conversely, patients with mild symptoms who ought to wait might be treated with cimetidine in a cost-ineffective way.

Accurate numbers are desperately needed to evaluate the cost-effectiveness of these alternative strategies. Dr. Frank Pancotto of Duke Medical School analyzed the yield from a series of 958 endoscopic examinations at their university hospital to which patients were referred from primary care physicians. Perhaps we can presume that these patients had already completed an unsuccessful therapeutic trial. Of this group, 10 had cancers; 182 had ulcers of which 139 were gastric; 117 had no detectable disease; and 649 had the milder diseases of gastritis, esophagitis, or duodenitis. Endoscopy has side effects and a mortality of one to two per thousand. These numbers are summarized in Figure 5, which elaborates on one branch of the larger decision tree in Figure 4. The alternative decisions shown in these trees have major cost implications.

TOTAL COST OF ULCER DISEASE BEFORE CIMETIDINE

Three estimates of the total costs of ulcer disease have been made for 1975 and are the target for reduction by improved therapy. The high-cost figure of $2.6 billion comes from a Stanford Research Institute (SRI) study,[51] the low-cost figure of $1.27 billion comes from the National Commission on Digestive Diseases,[52] and the midpoint estimate of $1.96 billion comes from Fineberg and Pearlman, who provide a lengthy critique of these cost estimates[46] (Table 2).

There is the problem of joint products that must be considered; that is, patients in hospitals are often treated for more than one disease. In the SRI study, mortality costs are based on lost earnings discounted at the rather low rate of 2½% per year. They, therefore, value the life of a 50- to 54-year-old man at $156,000 and a woman of similar age at

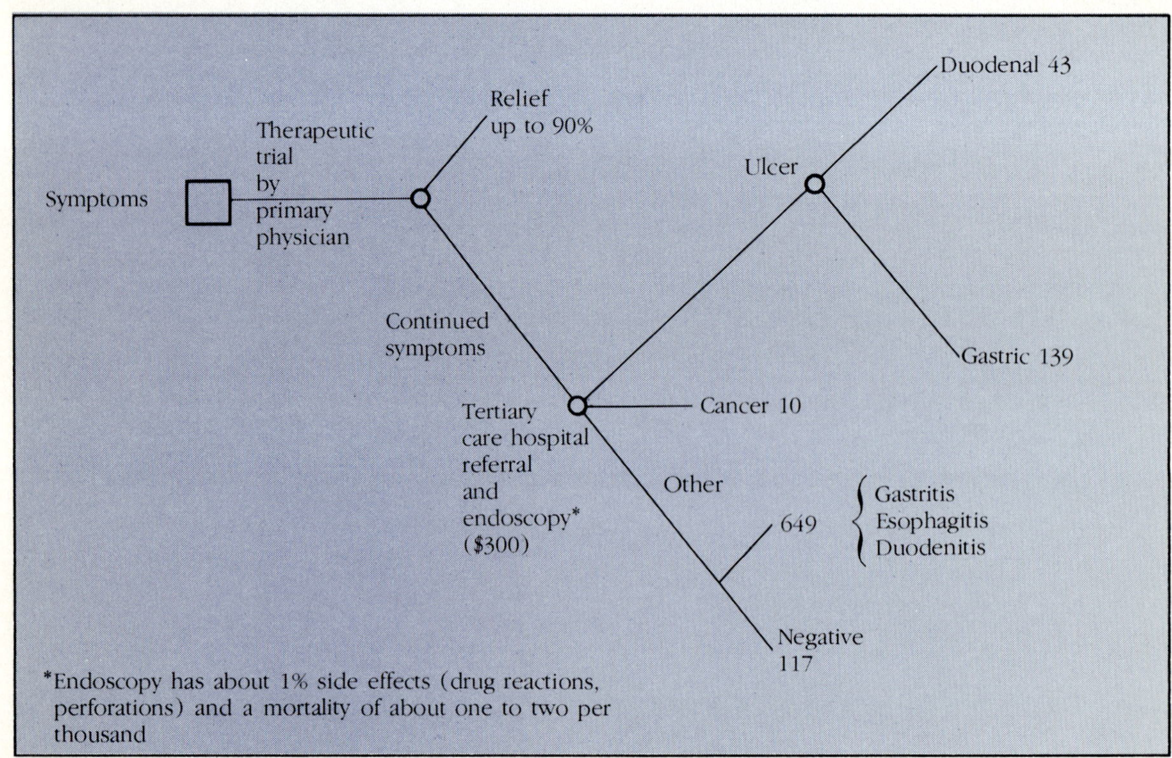

Figure 5. Yield from 958 endoscopy examinations at a tertiary care hospital (Source: Frank Pancotto, M.D.)

$111,000. Duodenal and gastric ulcer costs are not separated due to lack of information. Morbidity costs included the cost of worker absenteeism and the costs of care of the disabled who were not in the work force. Suffice it to say that the large differences in cost estimates reflect the lack of data, and the primitive state of this kind of analysis.

One of the interesting features of the cost-benefit literature on cimetidine is its sequencing. The first studies in the absence of data are based on expert opinion.[45] Later studies have actually analyzed experience, but were limited to patient populations for which appropriate data were available: Texas Medicaid patients,[53] surgical rates,[54,55] and household surveys in Rhode Island.[56]

Measuring the Change in Costs

To estimate the full magnitude of the cimetidine effect, one would like to measure all the component costs shown in Table 2 for the national population. However, this may require the crudest, most approximate measures. Greater accuracy has been achieved in studies that focus narrowly on a select population and specific components of the problem.

Pre-Cimetidine Averages Versus Projected Trend Lines

Several studies have reported a steadily declining number of operations and hospital discharges for both duodenal and gastric ulcer over the past 15 years. This decline has accelerated since the introduction of cimetidine. The long-run decline in hospital use prior to the introduction of cimetidine is somewhat puzzling but may be the result of antacid use or other variables. The question is which comparison should be the basis for study: the pre-cimetidine average of several years, or an extrapolation of the downward trend after 1977? Several studies are discussed below.

The Robinson Associates asked experts to project the changes that would occur if 80% of the duodenal ulcer population were to use cimetidine.[45] These estimates were then checked against information found in the literature, and the figures were recalculated accordingly. Duodenal ulcer costs, direct and indirect, were reduced from $2.192 billion to $1.547 billion, a 29% reduction. Applying this to all ulcer patients, the savings were 20%. What this approach gains in breadth, it may have sacrificed in accuracy.

Geweke and Weisbrod[53] analyzed the costs of medical care for 1200 Texas Medicaid duodenal ulcer patients before (without) and after (with) cimetidine treatment. Depending on the assumptions, the savings ranged from 11 to 63% of medical care costs. By considering a specific population, they were able to adjust statistically for patient characteristics; however, this population may not be representative of the country as a whole. Indirect costs were not considered.

Hospital use statistics, a household survey of ambulatory care, and records for a statewide workday loss insurance plan were used in Rhode Island.[51] One of the important aspects of this study is that it considered the use of cimetidine for patients without duodenal ulcer disease. Twenty-seven percent of cimetidine patients had a diagnosed gastric ulcer, and 29% had other or unspecified conditions. Projected regression lines for hospital and surgical use were the standard for comparison (a conservative test of the effect). The investigators found no change in hospital discharges or length of stay, but did find a significant decline in ulcer operations. The savings in hospital and physician costs ranged from 5 to 10%.

Table 2

Estimated Costs of Ulcer Disease in 1975
H. Fineberg and L. Pearlman
(millions of dollars)[46]

	National Commission on Digestive Diseases[52]	Stanford Research Institute[54]	Approximate midpoint estimates
Direct costs			
Hospitalization	$ 501	$ 803	$ 652
Physician visits	123	240	182
Drugs		100	
Nursing home care	102*	11	108*
Other professional		3	
Subtotal	726	1,157	942
Indirect costs†			
Mortality	369	357	369
Morbidity	179‡	1,116	648
Subtotal	548	1,473	1,017
Total	$1,274	$2,630	$1,959

*This sum represents the total for drugs, nursing homes, and other professional costs. Figures were not broken down further

†Future earnings discounted at 2.5 percent

‡This figure is imputed from information supplied in the NCDD report

The household survey found 59 cimetidine users and 85 noncimetidine respondents with ulcers; 27% of cimetidine users had gastric ulcers. "Since cimetidine is not approved by the Food and Drug Administration for the treatment of gastric ulcer, those reporting gastric ulcers were eliminated from both study groups."[53] Cimetidine users seemed to have better mental health (not statistically significant), less hospital use, and fewer disability days from all causes. There was greater compliance with cimetidine than for other medications. Annual costs were lower for cimetidine users ($310 to $409). According to the Rhode Island study, insurance claims fell from 1.987 per thousand in 1974 to 1.145 per thousand in 1979, for this group.

COMMENTS AND CONCLUSIONS

The cost-benefit and cost-effectiveness studies are consistent in their findings of reduced costs, improved outcome, and greatest benefits for cimetidine, although there were substantial differences in the magnitude of the savings. However, the following are still questions for deliberation: Why did the number of ulcer disease patients being treated in hospitals decline steadily before the introduction of cimetidine? What would have happened without it? What is the relative increase in benefits when cimetidine is compared with antacid use? Is cimetidine cost-effective for gastric ulcer? If not, what should be done about gastric ulcer patients now receiving cimetidine? Would any likely change in the numbers make physicians change their decisions with respect to cimetidine and duodenal ulcers? (This is called sensitivity analysis. One possible change is the discovery of a new, better, or less costly drug.) Do the major unanswered problems lie with the appropriate sequencing of tests and treatment, wait-and-see approach, upper GI series, endoscopy, or therapeutic trials? And finally, is it cost-effective for a large number of people who do not have duodenal ulcers to receive cimetidine?

Cimetidine as a model. When considering cimetidine as a model, concerns arise at a different level. Should cost-benefit analyses applied to cimetidine be advocated for a wide range of medical interventions? Would these analyses be useful for medical interventions where the evidence as to effectiveness is less clear and/or the benefits smaller and the costs higher? My answer is a guarded yes. Third party purchasers of medical care should be willing to demand some cost-benefit and/or cost-effectiveness evaluation before they agree to pay, in the same way that any large corporation inquires carefully about any large and repeated purchase it makes. If such demands are made, the evidence will be forthcoming. However, these analyses cannot withstand the scrutiny that could occur in a political-legislative battle or in a court of law.

Cimetidine provides one of the easiest cases to argue in favor of applying cost-benefit and cost-effectiveness analysis. Only very rarely will an easier example occur, such as with polio vaccine. Applying these analyses to other medical problems will not always be this easy. However, use of such analyses to deny the use of a particular therapy or payment for it will be nearly impossible. A consideration of the current turmoil about paying for abortions and Laetrile shows that these issues are debated on grounds other than scientific.

State Medicaid programs and private insurers may not make their decisions based solely on the kind of analyses described here. Some states might choose to spend Medicaid funds in order to support their medical-industrial complex, or they may be concerned with the effect of reduced absenteeism on state income taxes. Private insurers may be more concerned with their share of the health insurance market under competitive conditions. *Third parties* are not the only decision makers; *providers* of care have a different set of concerns. For some it is money, and for all it is the desire to be helpful and hopeful for their *patients*, who are another group of decision makers. There is a long list of cost-effective activities that most people reject or ignore. Cimetidine is special in that all three key decision makers "win." Therefore, the cost-benefit analyses are not disputed. This is why cimetidine as a model has limited applicability to all medical care. In short, for good or bad, right or wrong, societal costs and benefits are only one criterion for decision making.

Personally, I am delighted to see the effort that has gone into cimetidine evaluation. Hopefully, there will be more such efforts, but they won't answer all our problems.

REFERENCES

1. Hibbard P, Strom B: Unpublished Literature Review of Cimetidine Trials, University of Pennsylvania, Philadelphia, 1981
2. Blackwood WS et al: Cimetidine in duodenal ulcer. *Lancet* 2:174–176, 1976
3. Bodemar G, Walan A: Cimetidine in the treatment of active duodenal and prepyloric ulcers. *Lancet* 2:161–164, 1976
4. Bank S et al: Histamine H_2-receptor antagonists in the treatment of duodenal ulcers. *South African Medical Journal* 50:1781–1785, 1976
5. Gray GR et al: Oral cimetidine in severe duodenal ulceration. *Lancet* 1:4–7, 1977
6. Semb LS et al: A double-blind multicentre comparative study of cimetidine and placebo in short-term treatment of active

duodenal ulceration, in Burland WL, Simkins MA (eds): Cimetidine — Proceedings of the Second International Symposium on Histamine H$_2$-Receptor Antagonists. *Excerpta Medica*: 248-253, 1977

7. Northfield TC, Blackwood WS: Controlled clinical trial of cimetidine for duodenal ulcer, in Burland WL, Simkins MA (eds): Cimetidine — Proceedings of the Second International Symposium on Histamine H$_2$-Receptor Antagonists. *Excerpta Medica*: 272-273, 1977

8. Moshal MG et al: Treatment of duodenal ulcers with cimetidine. *South African Medical Journal* 52:760-763, 1977

9. Lambert R et al: Traitement de l'ulcere gastrique et duodenal par la cimetidine. *Gastroenterologie Clinique et Biologique* 1:855-860, 1977

10. Binder HJ et al: Cimetidine in the treatment of duodenal ulcer. *Gastroenterology* 74: 380-388, 1978

11. Villalobos JJ et al: Cimetidine in the treatment of duodenal ulcer: double-blind study. *Journal of International Medical Research* 6:351-354, 1978

12. Hetzel DJ et al: Cimetidine treatment of duodenal ulceration. *Gastroenterology* 74: 389-392, 1978

13. Gonvers JJ et al: Traitement de l'ulcere duodenal par la cimetidine. *Schweizerische Medizinische Wochenschrift* 108:1081-1083, 1978

14. Mazure PA et al: Cimetidina en el tratamiento de la ulcera duodenal activa. *Acta Gastroenterologica Latinoamericana* 8:17-28, 1978

15. Porro GB et al: Treatment of active duodenal ulcer with oral cimetidine: a multicenter controlled endoscopic trial. *Digestion* 17: 383-386, 1978

16. Peter P et al: Cimetidine for duodenal ulcer, in Creutzfeldt W (ed): Cimetidine—Proceedings of an International Symposium on Histamine H$_2$-Receptor Antagonists. *Excerpta Medica*: 190-201, 1978

17. Gilsanz V et al: Cimetidine for duodenal ulcer. *Lancet* 1:151, 1979

18. Bardham KD et al: Comparison of two doses of cimetidine and placebo in the treatment of duodenal ulcer: a multicentre trial. *Gut* 20: 68-74, 1979

19. Ubileuz R: Cimetidine in the treatment of active duodenal ulcer: a double-blind study. *Current Therapeutic Research* 25:243-250, 1979

20. Figueroa RB, Espejo HR: Cimetidine in active duodenal ulcer. *Current Therapeutic Research* 25:16-24, 1979

21. Hentschel VE et al: Die Behandlung des ulcus duodeni und des prapylorischen ulcus ventriculi mit Cimetidin. *Wiener Klinische Wochenschrift* 91:53-57, 1979

22. Matos-Villalobos M, Avella J: Ulcera duodenal: tratamiento doble ciego con cimetidina-placebo. *GEN* 33:39-43, 1979

23. Mazure PA et al: Cimetidine in active duodenal ulcer. *Current Therapeutic Research* 27:601-607, 1980

24. Bardham KD et al: Long-term treatment with cimetidine in duodenal ulceration. *Lancet* 1: 900-901, 1977

25. Porro GB, Petrillo M: Long-term treatment with cimetidine in duodenal ulceration. *Lancet* 1: 1366-1367, 1977

26. Gray GR et al: Long-term cimetidine in the management of severe duodenal ulcer dyspepsia. *Gastroenterology* 74:397-401, 1978

27. Blackwood WS et al: Prevention by bedtime cimetidine of duodenal-ulcer relapse. *Lancet* 1:626-627, 1978

28. Mekel RCPM: Long-term treatment with cimetidine. *South African Medical Journal* 54:1089-1091, 1978

29. Bardham KD et al: Double-blind comparison of cimetidine and placebo in the maintenance of healing of chronic duodenal ulceration. *Gut* 20: 158-162, 1979

30. Hetzel DJ et al: Prevention of duodenal ulcer relapse by cimetidine: a one-year double-blind trial. *Medical Journal of Austria* 1:529-531, 1979

31. Berstad A et al: Maintenance treatment of duodenal ulcer patients with a single bedtime dose of cimetidine. *Scandinavian Journal of Gastroenterology* 14: 827-831, 1979

32. Dronfield MW et al: Controlled trial of maintenance cimetidine treatment in healed duodenal ulcer: short and long-term effects. *Gut* 20:526-530, 1979

33. Sonnenberg A et al: Rezidivprophylaxe des ulcus duodeni mit Cimetidin. *Deutsche Medizinische Wochenschrift* 104:725, 730, 1979

34. Burland WL et al: Cimetidine treatment for the prevention of recurrence of duodenal ulcer: an international collaborative study. *Postgraduate Medical Journal* 56:173-176, 1980

35. Korman MG et al: Relapse rate of duodenal ulcer after cessation of long-term cimetidine treatment. *Digestive Diseases and Sciences* 25:88-91, 1980

36. Bodemar G, Walan A: Two-year follow-up after one year's treatment with cimetidine or placebo. *Lancet* 1:38-39, 1980

37. Beecher HK: The powerful placebo. *Journal of the American Medical Association* 159:1602-1606, 1955

38. Frank J: *Persuasion and Healing*, Baltimore, Johns Hopkins, revised edition, 1973, ch 6

39. Piper DW: The treatment of chronic peptic ulcer. *Gastrointestinal Research* 6:109-125, 1980

40. Ippoliti AF et al: Cimetidine versus intensive antacid therapy for duodenal ulcer. *Gastroenterology* 74:393-395, 1978

41. Fedeli G et al: A controlled study comparing cimetidine treatment to an intensive antacid regimen in the therapy of uncomplicated duodenal ulcer. *Digestive Diseases and Sciences* 24:758-762, 1979

42. Malchow H et al: Cimetidin in der stationären Behandlung des peptischen Ulkus. *Deutsch Medizinische Wocheschrift* 103:149-152, 1978

43. Hollander D, Harlan J: Antacids versus placebos in peptic ulcer therapy. *Journal of the American Medical Association* 226: 1181-1185, 1973

44. Peterson WL et al: Healing of duodenal ulcer with an antacid regimen. *New England Journal of Medicine* 297:341-345, 1977

45. Robinson Associates: The Impact of Cimetidine on the National Cost of Duodenal Ulcers. Bryn Mawr, Pennsylvania, Unpublished Report, 1978

46. Fineberg H, Pearlman L: Benefit and Cost Analysis of Medical Interventions: The Case of Cimetidine and Peptic Ulcer Disease. *United States Congress, Office of Technology Assessment*, Washington, DC, 1981

47. Bader J et al: Treatment of gastric ulcer by cimetidine. A multicentre trial, in Burland WL, Simkins MA (eds): Cimetidine: Proceedings of the Second International Symposium on Histamine H$_2$-Receptor Antagonists, *Excerpta Medica*: 287-292, 1977

48. Ciclitira PJ et al: A controlled trial of cimetidine in the treatment of gastric ulcer, in Burland WL, Simkins MA (eds): Cimetidine: Proceedings of the Second International Symposium on Histamine H$_2$-Receptor Antagonists, *Excerpta Medica*: 283-286, 1977

49. Dyck WP et al: Cimetidine and placebo in the treatment of benign gastric ulcer. A multicenter double blind study. *Gastroenterology* 74:410-415, 1978

50. Frost F et al: Cimetidine in patients with gastric ulcer: a multicentre controlled trial. *British Medical Journal* 2:795-797, 1977

51. von Haunalter G, Chandler VV: *Cost of Ulcer Disease in the United States.* Menlo Park, California, Stanford Research Institute, February, 1977

52. Almy TP et al: Report of the Workgroup on the Socioeconomic Impact of Digestive Diseases of the Subcommittee on Epidemiology and Impact. *Report to the*

Congress of the United States of the National Commission on Digestive Diseases, DHEW Publication No. (N1+) 79–1887, 4:249–338, 1979

53. Geweke JR, Weisbrod A: Some economic consequences of technological advance in medical care: the case of a new drug, in Helms RB (ed): *Drugs and Health*. Washington, DC, American Enterprise Institute for Public Policy Research, 1981, pp 235–271

54. Fineberg H, Pearlman L: Surgical treatment of peptic ulcer in the United States. *Lancet* 1:1305–1307, 1981

55. Wyllie JH et al: Effect of cimetidine on surgery for duodenal ulcer. *Lancet* 1:1307–1308, 1981

56. Rhode Island Health Services Research Inc: The Effect of Cimetidine on Peptic Ulcer Disease in Rhode Island. Providence, Rhode Island, RIHSR, July 1981

Discussion

Question: Is there a way of clearly separating in advance patients who are likely to benefit more by a drug, such as cimetidine?

Response: Physicians often use a drug, such as cimetidine, without any objective evidence of the specific disease they are treating. If they used good information, then the response would be more positive than if the drug were used simply for nondescript pain.

Response: We looked at four options in treating people with symptoms of dyspepsia. We didn't start with ulcer disease because patients don't present with ulcers, but rather with symptoms. The clinician's problem is whether to treat patients symptomatically with less than full ulcer therapy, perhaps just a placebo or small doses of antacids, or treat them with cimetidine four times a day. Another option would be a thorough work-up. Usually the first choice is an upper GI x-ray. Within that realm, two options are available: 1) appropriately treating the condition noted on the upper GI x-ray or 2) continuing with an upper GI endoscopy for people who show gastric ulcer on the upper GI x-ray. This poses a major diagnostic issue: The readings of the upper GI series might be misleading because of the confusion between gastric ulcer and gastric cancer. But the two important clinical questions are whether to treat people for dyspepsia or to treat them with cimetidine without looking for ulcer on upper GI x-ray or endoscopy. The possibility is that one might miss a gastric cancer. This, however, may not be an important reason not to prescribe cimetidine immediately since it is not clear whether waiting 6 or 12 weeks to diagnose a gastric cancer is harmful. If there were reason to think that it might be harmful to wait, we would like to avoid that, but in many cases you might simply postpone telling a patient the bad news without changing mortality.

The other issue is whether cimetidine works for people who don't have duodenal or gastric ulcer. Part of the problem with that question is the poor relationship between symptoms of true duodenal ulcer disease and the presence of duodenal ulcer. Cimetidine appeared at a fortuitous time, as endoscopy had also become available to evaluate ulcer disease. That may be one reason for the many cimetidine studies, since a procedure was now available to study the disease and its course. It may be that many people who did not have a diagnosed duodenal ulcer and who participated in the studies did indeed have duodenal ulcer disease, but did not have a duodenal ulcer at the time. In other words, many people who do not have that diagnosis may well have the disease and will benefit from the drug. Thus, it looks as if cimetidine may reduce mortality and that there may be some positive cost benefit in providing it for people with nonulcer dyspepsia.

Dr. Neuhauser: The key is that the decision rules are going to be rather complicated and subtle and not the kind that are easily addressed by a simple regulation by a third-party payer. So this type of broad-ranging decision is going to pose problems with the third-party payers. To write regulations that follow exactly the set of decision roles may be exceedingly difficult and even if possible may be ignored altogether.

Question: What should be the role of postmarketing surveillance in cost-effectiveness study in other areas?

Dr. Neuhauser: One is keeping track of potential side effects that may occur. I was struck with the drug company's genuine effort to do this. Another may be how the drug is being used, for whom, and why. The drug companies and the decision makers should work closely in generating or collecting information that would fit into the decision model.

Response: I was a bit disturbed by a reference to coronary bypass surgery reimbursement based on the fact that both the physician and the patient might benefit. The third party, of course, is the loser. Now, a third-party reimburser, it seems to me, should consider the net benefits to the consumer. In this case, as far as I know, mortality outcome has not been proven to be much greater. On the other hand, patients believe they benefit, and that is why they want it paid for. Now this concerns a large amount of money in public policy decision making and I'm puzzled as to how you actually reached a conclusion.

Dr. Neuhauser: Quite a few third parties are not clear on the cost-benefit effects of their various decisions. One of the bureaucratic fallbacks is to simply look at how much money is being spent, rather than at the total net impact on society as a whole. In the absence of that information, which is acceptable and easily available to third-party decision makers, it may be too easy to say how much revenue we have got, how much money we are spending, and how we can cope with that. We may, however, fall a bit short of that ideal. Even if third-party payers had this information, it is not altogether clear to me that they would use it. Perhaps they are more concerned with their share of the market and their competition with other third-party payers in the area. If they can add this as a benefit, whether it is cost effective or not in terms of a formal societal analysis, they may well go ahead and do it. So, in terms of the business analysis of their strategy, even if they had the cost-benefit analysis, they may set it aside and decide that, if they can get the contract, even if it means adding something of little value, they will go ahead and do it. I suppose this level of cost-benefit analysis carefully measures patient preferences, rather than contribution to society as a whole.

In the case of cimetidine and deductibles, cimetidine, even for the most appropriate category of patients for which we could decide it is cost beneficial, is likely to be eliminated from the deductible. The $300 endoscopy, which may be appropriate for a small number of patients, will be covered.

Medical Technology Decision Making in a Political Environment at the Federal Level

Joyce C. Lashof, M.D.

Dean, School of Public Health
University of California
Berkeley, California

Government policies toward the development and diffusion of medical technology date back to the turn of the 20th century. They have slowly evolved from initial concern with the honest labeling of drugs to the present emphasis on safety, efficacy and cost of all medical technology.

The evolution of government policy toward medical technology is closely related to the increasing complexity of technology and of the organization of society, including changing views on the role of government. In the early 1900s there were only a dozen useful drugs and little else of importance in medical therapy, whereas in the 1980s medical care is dominated by high technology. In 1906, the only relevant law was the Food and Drug Act that prohibited mislabeling; today all aspects of technology from development through evaluation, diffusion, and use are affected by government agencies, laws, or regulations. A brief review of these elements will be given in this paper.

OFFICE OF TECHNOLOGY ASSESSMENT

Established by law in 1972 and governed by a Congressional Board of six representatives and six senators, equally divided by party, the Office of Technology Assessment (OTA) is charged with providing to the Congress "early indications of the probable beneficial and adverse impacts of the applications of technology." In response to this task, the Health Program of OTA carries out studies dealing with the development of medical technology and the assessment of its safety, efficacy, and cost effectiveness in making decisions regarding resource allocation. I will refer to several of these studies in the course of this discussion.

In general, OTA reports to Congress emphasize general policy implications rather than conclusions concerning specific technologies, and its assessments review individual technologies only as case studies to illustrate major policy issues.

MAJOR FEDERAL AGENCIES AND LAWS AFFECTING MEDICAL TECHNOLOGY

The primary Federal agency stimulating development of medical technology through support of basic research is the National Institutes of Health (NIH). It is becoming increasingly involved, however, in evaluation of efficacy. Most recently, through consensus conferences often conducted in conjunction with the National Center for Health Care Technology, NIH has begun to address economic, social, and ethical issues related to medical technology use.

The Food and Drug Administration (FDA) is the primary agency responsible for assuring the safety and efficacy of drugs and devices, thus controlling at least their initial marketing. The diffusion of expensive technologies is also affected by the Health Planning Law, 93-641r, primarily through the state certificate of need requirements. The appropriateness of use of medical procedures including hospitalization, surgical intervention, and laboratory testing is the concern of PSRO. Finally, reimbursement decisions under Medicare and Medicaid also have an impact on the use of medical technology.

National Center for Health Care Technology

In an effort to coordinate these activities and provide a focus for federal technology assessment, the National Center for Health Care Technology (NCHCT) was established in 1978. The legislation establishing the center charged it with four major responsibilities:

• To undertake and support medical technology assessments that address issues of safety, effectiveness, cost effectiveness, and social and ethical impacts.

• To support studies of the factors that affect the use of medical technologies and of methods for disseminating information about these technologies.

• To encourage and support evaluations of safety and efficacy of selected new and old technologies. When appropriate and practical, the center is to develop and disseminate exemplary norms, standards, and criteria concerning the use of the health care technologies that it has studied.

• To make recommendations to the Health Care Financing Administration (HCFA) regarding policies on Federal reimbursement for the use of medical technologies.

NCHCT has made progress in carrying out these functions and, in July, 1981, Congress authorized its continuation. The fiscal 1982 budget, however, provides no funding for the center, although it calls specifically for allocation of some of the funds of the National Center for Health Services Research to certain assessment and reimbursement advice functions of NCHCT.

National Center for Health Services Research

The National Center for Health Services Research (NCHSR) was established in 1968 to conduct research in organization and financing of health care, health manpower, and the evaluation of quality of medical care. The current budget cuts, coupled with the earmarking of almost a third of NCHSR funds to the previous responsibilities of the NCHCT, however, make it difficult to predict just what activities NCHSR will be able to undertake in the coming years.

30

ACUTE INFORMATION NEEDS

With the specific role of each agency being less clear today, the need for information relevant to implementation of the general mandate for technology assessment becomes particularly acute. It is becoming increasingly clear, however, that only a fraction of that information is easily accessible. As we review all of these agencies and laws, it is apparent that the type of information needed and the responsibility for obtaining that information and translating it into policy decisions depend on the mandate of each agency and on the current concept of the role of government.

RETROSPECT ON U.S. DRUG LAW

A brief review of the history of U.S. drug law illustrates this graphically. The 1906 Food and Drug Law contained the injunction that labels not be "false or misleading in any particular." The Supreme Court, however, ruled that these requirements related only to the composition of the drug and not to claims of therapeutic efficacy.

The reasoning of the court is especially relevant. Chief Justice Holmes, speaking for the court, based his opinion on the fact that Congress did not mean "to distort the uses of constitutional power to establishing criteria in regions where opinions are far apart." The decision was thus based on the court's opinion that the state of knowledge was not adequate to reach a conclusion concerning the efficacy of a drug.

The governmental philosophy at that time was that the market system was the best protector of the consumer and that government should act only where the consumer could not. Since the consumer could not carry out the tests necessary to determine the composition of a drug, such testing was the rightful responsibility of government. The consumer, however, was considered capable of deciding whether or not a drug was effective.[1] This approach held sway until 1938. By that time, however, new drugs were developed with greater therapeutic effect, but also with greater toxicity. FDA took the position that the safe use of such drugs required more knowledge than a consumer could be expected to have. Thus, the 1938 Drug Law, responsive to these changes in technology, prohibited the sale of unsafe drugs and required specific instructions on labels.

On the belief that certain drugs were only safe when used following a careful diagnosis and under the direction of a physician, the FDA proceeded to promulgate regulations requiring some drugs to be dispensed only upon a physician's prescription.

Thus, the doctor's judgment came to supplant that of the consumer. These regulations were incorporated into law by the Humphrey-Dunham amendments of 1951. It was not until 1962, however, that the issue of efficacy was addressed. By the 1960s, scientific advances had introduced a much larger number of potent and potentially toxic drugs, for which the mechanisms of action and indications of use required thorough testing and evaluation. It was no longer believed possible for the physician in practice to evaluate the efficacy of a drug.

The 1962 Drug Law substituted the findings of experts for the judgment of physicians. The new law added three requirements:

- Substantial evidence of effectiveness of the drug was to be shown.
- Affirmative action by the FDA had to be taken prior to marketing.
- FDA was given jurisdiction over testing.

Current FDA regulatory policy based on this law has evolved in response to court actions. By 1970, the current testing requirements were promulgated and informal clinical evidence, even by experts, was no longer considered meeting the "substantial evidence of effectiveness" provision of the 1962 law.[1]

CONCERN FOR COST-EFFECTIVENESS

Government responsibility for assuring the consumer of the safety and efficacy of drugs by the use of the best scientific methodology is now firmly accepted. Even in the current antiregulatory climate this responsibility of FDA is not challenged. We can thus expect efforts towards streamlining rather than dismantling the drug approval process.[2]

Beyond safety and efficacy, there is appearing now a new concern for cost. During the latter part of the 1970s, the term "cost effectiveness" became a "buzz word" both in the Congressional and executive branches of government. With the rising cost of medical care, much of which has been blamed, rightly or wrongly, on increases in the use of medical technology, it was only natural that the techniques of cost-effectiveness analysis (CEA) and cost-benefit analysis (CBA) were applied to the health field.

APPLICABILITY OF COST CRITERIA BY FDA

The applicability of CEA/CBA by FDA to the drug approval process is problematic. Such criteria are not referred to in the law and the direct application of CEA in approval or denial of a "New Drug Application" (NDA) would certainly be subject to legal challenge. However, indirect use of some economic criteria can and does influence the FDA drug approval process.

Approval Priority Rating

FDA sets priorities for its review of new drugs according to potential therapeutic usefulness. Drugs are rated according to their newness on a scale of 1 to 6 and their therapeutic advantage on a scale of A to C. For example, an entirely new molecular entity that offers a major therapeutic advantage would be rated 1A, whereas an already marketed drug which offers no appreciable therapeutic advantage and for which approval is sought for a new use would be rated 6C.[3] The criteria used for such a priority rating are based on scientific data on safety and efficacy, but the economic implications of a 1A drug are clear. Any drug that shows a marked therapeutic advantage leading to decreased hospitalization and morbidity is ostensibly more cost effective than the existing treatment, and it does not require sophisticated cost-effectiveness analysis to prove this. Although the economic impact was not FDA's prime motivation in developing the priority classification, a drug with a 1A classification will receive expeditious review rather than wait for its turn in the pipeline. NDAs for 1A and 1B drugs must contain all the safety and efficacy data required for any NDA. On a rare occasion, however, FDA may accept less long-term safety data for an exceptional 1A drug, sometimes obligating the manufacturer to conduct post marketing surveillance.[4] In the absence of therapeutic advantage, however, economic arguments have not been used in developing the priority classification.

Theoretically, a new drug with no therapeutic advantage but less expensive than current drugs could be given priority consideration in the review process. An adequate evaluation of the cost effectiveness of early approval of such a drug would, however, require calculating the costs of delayed approval of other drugs in the pipeline that would be bumped. This does not seem feasible.

In its review of CEA, OTA analyzed the effects if cost-effectiveness analysis was actually added as a criterion for market approval. A simplistic model was developed to illustrate the type of data needed. To compare four treatments for the same disease, it would be necessary to determine the safety and efficacy of each agent and translate it into a health effect unit. Decreased morbidity and mortality would be a positive health effect while side effects and adverse reactions would be negative health effects. These effects would have to be translated into measurable units to calculate a "net health effect." To calculate costs, one would need to know the costs of purchasing the drug, the cost of treating drug-induced side effects, and possibly the costs of treating other illnesses among the persons whose lives are saved. This latter cost is the subject of strong controversy among economists and CEA methodologists with no agreement in sight.

The cost-effectiveness (CE) ratio would thus be the net cost per unit of net health effect. After calculating the CE ratio for each of a number of treatments, a determination would be required as to how much more cost effective a treatment needs to be for market approval to be granted. By whom and how such a decision should be made is speculative.

OTA discussions with consumer advocates, FDA employees, and representatives of the pharmaceutical industry revealed general agreement that cost-effectiveness analysis is not an appropriate criterion in the process of approval of drugs and medical devices. A number of problems were identified, and key prominence was given to these issues:

- Adequate cost estimates of treating illnesses using alternative forms of therapy are lacking and it would be difficult to generate the relevant data bases.

- The price of a drug or device is neither known to FDA, nor subject to FDA approval at time of marketing and, even if known, could change over time.

- Finally, the cost of carrying out such studies may inhibit innovation. Besides, the cost-effectiveness of drug or device is markedly influenced by conditions of its use such as dosage regimen, patient acceptability, and indications, all of which might change over time.[5]

ROLE OF ECONOMIC FACTORS IN FDA DECISIONS

The regulatory burden imposed by a CBA/CEA requirement would be heavy, and certainly not in keeping with the current political mood. This is not to say that economic considerations play no part in FDA's decisions or in Congressional reaction they evoke. Two examples may be cited.

Ban on Diethylstilbestrol (DES)

Based on its finding that DES is a carcinogenic substance, FDA, in 1972, moved to ban the use of DES in animal feed. Legal proceedings to prevent the ban were undertaken by the livestock industry, which since 1965 had depended on DES to increase muscle and fat content of animals and reduce cost of meat and poultry production. In responding to the court challenges, FDA, in 1976, issued a statement on potential inflationary impact of the ban. FDA maintained that the impact would be minimal, resulting in no more than a $2 to $3 annual cost increase per consumer. These data were challenged by the livestock industry. Congressional hearings were held, court challenges continued, and it was not until 1979 that Commissioner Kennedy successfully ordered the withdrawal of DES. At that time, the Commissioner stated:

> FDA is not authorized, under the Food, Drug and Cosmetic Act, in considering the question of whether a new animal drug has been shown to be safe for use, to weigh the "socio-economic" benefits that that drug provides against a health risk to the ultimate human consumers of treated animals. Even were I to attempt to weigh the benefits of DES against its risks, this record would not provide sufficient information to compute the risk associated with DES or to determine whether, and to what extent, use of DES provides any health benefit or even any economic benefit to society.[6]

Use of Antibiotics in Animal Feed

The other, somewhat related example is the continuing controversy over the use of antibiotics in animal feed. Antibacterial agents have been used in animal feed to prevent disease, promote growth, and improve feed efficiency since the early 1950s. By the late 1960s, concern was expressed regarding the impact of the widespread use of antibiotics in animals and humans on the development of drug-resistant bacteria. By 1977, the FDA moved to ban the use of penicillin and restrict the use of tetracycline in animal feed premixes. The agricultural industry protested the proposed regulation on economic grounds and carried their case to Congress. The Office of Technology Assessment and the National Academy of Sciences, upon requests of Congress, have studied the issue and numerous Congressional hearings have been held.[7-9]

After reviewing the data on the potential risk to human health and the data on the economic impact of the proposed restrictions, OTA stated among other things that:

> The trade-off is therefore between immediate economic benefits and future health risks. These decisions involve value judgment and

cannot be based simply on monetary considerations. And the lack of scientific certainty on the magnitude of both the probable health risk and the attributed increases in meat production makes the formulation of a balance-sheet approach difficult. [7]

Since under current law the FDA cannot consider the economic impact of restricting these drugs, it has the responsibility to act. Congress, however, responding to the concerns of the agricultural and pharmaceutical industries, has enacted legislation prohibiting the FDA from acting and has called for further study. Thus, when Congress feels that economic considerations are overriding, it does not hesitate to act.

FEDERAL HEALTH PROGRAM AS TOOL OF COST CONTROL

In essence, current FDA law reflects both our scientific ability to evaluate the safety and efficacy of drugs and a societal conviction that the complexity of such evaluation is beyond that of the consumer and is thus the province of government. The point at which we will feel that our ability to determine cost effectiveness is so solid, and yet not responsive enough to market forces, that we will move to incorporate such determination into FDA regulatory policy is hard to predict.

Nevertheless, cost-effectiveness analysis is receiving increasing attention in other governmental health programs and laws. Reimbursement decisions under Medicare and the PSRO program are the two most likely candidates for the use of data obtained from cost-benefit and cost-effectiveness analyses. Most recently, Congress, acting upon the report on cost effectiveness of pneumococcal vaccine, added coverage for its use under Medicare, while also requesting that OTA carry out a similar study for influenza vaccine. Congress is also pushing for data on cost effectiveness of psychotherapy and other mental health treatments before deciding on further coverage for psychiatric care.

At the same time, HCFA and the Public Health Service (PHS), formerly through NCHCT and now presumably through NCHSR, are refining their procedures for making reimbursement decisions under Medicare. The Social Security Act mandates that the Medicare Program shall pay only for services which are "reasonable and necessary" for diagnoses, treatment, or improved functioning. Generally, this has been applied to mean that once a procedure has moved from experimental status and is accepted by the local community it is "deemed reasonable and necessary." This decision is usually made locally, but when a coverage question is referred to the central HCFA office, it in turn requests a recommendation from the Public Health Service. The PHS has traditionally applied four criteria to coverage recommendations: safety, efficacy, state of development, and acceptance by the medical community. These recommendations generally have not attempted to specify indications for use—a function left to PSRO. HCFA did, however, set precedent in the case of the CT body scan decision by restricting coverage to uses supported by current evidence of efficacy.

Both HCFA and PHS are, however, considering a number of changes in the coverage process. HCFA is considering several actions, including issuing new guidelines that relate coverage to appropriate indications for use, utilizing cost as a criterion. Also, the National Center for Health Care Technology was considering utilizing three additional criteria in making its recommendations to HCFA, namely, conformity to health planning guidelines, relative efficacy, and cost effectiveness. The methodological problems faced in applying the last two criteria are extensive.

Reimbursement for Heart Transplants

Some of these problems are illustrated by the decision concerning payment for heart transplants. The issue was raised by Stanford University and referred by the HCFA regional office to the HCFA central office. HCFA requested advice from the NCHCT. Although noting that costs for the procedure were substantial, the NCHCT, in November, 1979, upon an analysis of safety and efficacy, recommended reimbursement for the procedure when carried out at Stanford, and so notified the university.

The Office of Health Regulation in HCFA, however, undertook a preliminary cost-effectiveness analysis and the Office of the Secretary of HHS requested a thorough review of the decision. At the same time, an administrative law judge in Arizona held that if Stanford was to be reimbursed, so too were other institutions.

Finally, in June of 1980, the Secretary decided to end regular reimbursement of heart transplants and, instead, to fund a study to analyze not only the medical safety and efficacy of transplantation, but also the social, economic, and ethical implications of a decision to reimburse for this procedure. This information is from Reiss JB et al (unpublished paper prepared for OTA). It is likely that this type of analysis will be undertaken in the future for newly introduced, equally expensive technologies.

It should also be noted that the PSRO program was enacted to assure that health services under Medicare and Medicaid are provided at the most economic level consistent with quality care. Although cost-effectiveness criteria have not been explicitly incorporated into standards of care, it appears possible for a PSRO to do so. It may not be practical for an individual PSRO to carry out sophisticated CEA studies, but it could keep physicians aware of the results of such studies, and thus influence physician behavior.

CURRENT GOVERNMENT STAND

The current administration believes that, by moving toward a competitive health care system, we will be able to do away with such Federal programs as PSRO and health planning but still control costs. Thus far, the government has been unable, or unwilling, to reach a decision as to whether or how resources for medical care should be limited and allocated. Some view the competitive market approach as a way of shifting the burden of resource allocation, especially regarding medical technology, from the government to the consumer. Who will support the research needed for informed decision making and how that information will be provided to the consumer remains to be seen.

Regardless of where or by whom the decisions will be made, our need for solid data based on well controlled studies will continue to grow. A complex, technologically advanced society cannot make decisions without an adequate understanding of their potential impact.

REFERENCES

1. Temin P: *Taking Your Medicine.* Cambridge, Mass, Harvard University Press, 1980
2. Demkovich LE: The FDA's new boss finds regulation "absolutely essential"—sometimes. *National Journal,* August 29, 1981
3. *New Drugs Evaluation Project: Briefing Book.* Rockville, Md, Food and Drug Administration, DHEW; October 1979
4. Cenerwall BS, Criqui MH: Prevention of the Wernicke-Korsakoff Syndrome: An updated cost-benefit analysis. *New England Journal of Medicine* 300:320, 1979
5. *The Implications of Cost-Effectiveness Analysis of Medical Technology,* GPO Stock No 052-003-00765-7. US Congress, Office of Technology Assessment, August 1980, pp 92-95
6. Diethylstilbestrol: Withdrawal of Approval of New Animal Drug Applications; Commissioner Decision. *Federal Register* 44:54900, September 21, 1979
7. *Drugs in Livestock Feed, Vol. I,* Technical Report, GPO Stock No 052-003-00685 US Congress, Office of Technology Assessment, June 1979
8. National Academy of Sciences, Committee to Study the Human Health Effects of Subtherapeutic Antibiotic Use in Animal Feeds: *The Effects on Human Health of Subtherapeutic Use of Antimicrobials in Animal Feeds.* Washington, DC, NAS, 1980
9. *Antibiotics in Animal Feed,* hearings before the Subcommittee on Health and Environment of the Committee on Interstate and Foreign Commerce, US House of Representatives, Washington, DC, June 1980. Washington, DC, US Government Printing Office, 1980

Discussion

APPROVED VS NONAPPROVED INDICATIONS

Question: Dr. Lashof indicated that the FDA has an important role in evaluating new drugs. Nevertheless, Dr. Neuhauser suggested that cimetidine was being prescribed for non-FDA approved uses. How can those two positions be reconciled?

Dr. Lashof: I am not sure I see the problem in terms of the FDA's role. The FDA approves a drug for its safety and efficacy and then outlines the approved use. The question then becomes: Does the FDA have a role in policing how a drug is used? If so, how could the FDA possibly enforce a physician's following the approved prescription? We have depended essentially on the canons of practice; PSROs now look at how physicians practice. If a physician uses a drug for a non-FDA approved indication and the patient brings a malpractice suit, the fact that the drug was prescribed for a nonapproved use may weigh heavily against the physician. That is the way the system currently operates.

Question: I am currently involved in the economic analysis of cimetidine in the long-run, and eventually wish to extrapolate to society the benefits resulting from multicenter trials. Clinicians prescribing cimetidine for nonapproved uses results in an adverse item that must be subtracted to obtain a net benefit. I presume there must be some medical benefits from nonapproved prescribing. In addition, new uses of old drugs have been discovered serendipitously. What are the clinical or health benefits from prescribing cimetidine for uses other than duodenal ulcer?

Response: Some well-documented research has shown the advantages of cimetidine over certain other agents, specifically in treating esophagitis. Since the literature indicates that cimetidine has been efficacious in relieving symptoms of esophagitis, many physicians use the drug for this condition. I do not know whether the evidence has definitely shown that there has been a histological improvement or if there has been endoscopic evidence that these patients have improved, but certainly symptoms improve dramatically. In other indications, such as dyspepsia, in the broad use of the term, most research has shown no significant improvement if a patient uses placebo versus cimetidine. Gastritis patients have not been shown to benefit from cimetidine usage. Physicians basically tend to rely on the literature and prescribe accordingly.

Response: We are not always operating in murky waters. Several sources provide clinicians with information. A drug company, as in the case of cimetidine, submits to the FDA the results of many studies for which indications were not approved. Data are also available in the literature. Thirdly, once a drug is available, other investigators may study it for other conditions and publish their findings.

Response: Two recently published papers discuss nonapproved uses. One deals with an antiandrogenic effect of cimetidine as a depilatory for women and a second indicates that cimetidine lowers parathormone levels.

Dr. Lashof: Do you know of a fair number of instances in which effective drug benefits have occurred serendipitously? Does this happen frequently or is it a rare phenomenon?

Response: I have not looked at this issue formally, but it seems that a lot of uses of drugs that are considered efficacious are not approved. A good example may be diphenylhydantoin, which is known to be a good antiarrhythmic in some situations, as is propranolol. There is no question that technologies can be useful for many things they were not originally tested for. The problem is that it becomes difficult to obtain evidence, because nobody is willing to pay for it. The manufacturers have no incentive to fund the studies for that sort of thing because the objective is just getting the drug on the market. People can adopt it knowing they can be reimbursed for it once they do adopt it.

Response: In terms of unapproved uses, in a study that is now completed but has not been published, we looked at the 100 most common drug uses, that is, drug indication pairs in the United States as defined by data from IMS. Although I do not remember the exact number, something on the order of 10 to 20% of those drug uses were unapproved; of those, about half have significant study data showing that they are efficacious. So unapproved uses are common and many are appropriate. We wrote to both pharmaceutical manufacturers and to the FDA to find out what studies had been undertaken prior to marketing. Somewhat to our surprise, about 80% of drugs were studied in relation to other drugs prior to marketing.

A lot of those studies were of antibiotics and antineoplastics, drugs that would be especially unethical to study relative to other active agents. The FDA, however, seems to be requiring studies of absolute efficacy for gastrointestinal and antiulcer drugs. Unlike the antibiotics and antitumor drugs, neither cimetidine nor antacids have been shown to change the natural history of the disease, although they may promote short-term healing. Thus, a study of absolute efficacy is not as unethical as it would be in the case of an antibiotic or an antitumor drug. In addition, to study relative efficacy of cimetidine versus a new H_2 blocker would require a large sample size, would be extremely expensive, and would be difficult to determine small differences in efficacy. The usual premarketing efficacy study of tens to hundreds of patients would not be sensitive enough to pick up a lack of efficacy in a new drug. Thus, the new drug would have to be tested against a placebo to study its efficacy.

Response: We have identified two major points. First, who makes the decisions for whom, and second, that of efficacy versus effectiveness. But the system we have today really doesn't work well in terms of separating these two decisions. For the developer of a drug, the incentive is to obtain approval. When this is granted, they know that physicians will also use it for nonapproved indications. Thus, once the drug has been approved for the initial indication, there is no incentive for the drug developer to spend the considerable amounts of money needed to prove efficacy for other indications. I do not think that malpractice in this area is common. I do not know of any malpractice cases in which a drug commonly used as accepted medical therapy for an approved indication is also used for a nonapproved indication. Propranolol, for instance, was initially approved for treating hypertension, but it has also been used to treat angina, which has only recently been approved. If a drug is commonly used, that may take precedence in a courtroom over what the FDA may have approved. Obviously physicians don't see that as a strong threat, because many indications for major drugs are recognized as being therapeutically efficacious in the general medical community, even though they have not been approved for those indications.

How can we make these decisions on medical technology without information? Nobody is doing the studies because there is no money in it, except possibly for the regulatory agencies and reimbursing parties, which basically means the Federal government. Until the information becomes available, I do not see how we are going to be able to answer the question about the marginal impacts of drugs.

Question: I would expect that cimetidine is probably the mark on the wall concerning the treatment of duodenal ulcer. If we are to continue developing new drugs, why does the FDA insist that we compare these with a placebo? That raises moral issues as well as cost effectiveness.

Dr. Lashof: The ethical question is can you hold a clinical trial on a new drug by comparing it with a placebo when you have an effective drug on the market? You would have great difficulty ethically looking at a new drug, but the law does not allow the FDA to look at relative efficacy as a criterion for drug approval.

Medical Technology Decision Making in a Political Environment at the State Level

Myrle A. Myers, R.Ph., M.S.

Chief, Pharmacy and Ambulatory Care Service
Division of Medical Assistance
Colorado Department of Social Services
Denver, Colorado

INTRODUCTION

The general characteristics of decision making in public arenas are not the same as those of the private sector. Decision making in private business is oriented toward maximizing profit. This is not always true for public programs, particularly those affecting the health of a recipient group. Emotional and moral issues, which may not enter into the cost-effectiveness equation, become an integral part of the decision-making process.

The number of people involved in private sector decisions is much smaller than those involved in public policymaking. Medical policies for public assistance programs are formulated at all levels of government. In addition, a wide range of groups participate in policy formation, including health professionals; state legislators; program administrators at both the federal and state levels; groups purporting to represent the general public, recipient rights, and taxpayers' rights; and other miscellaneous special interest groups.

Although medical technology decision making contains features that encompass cost-benefit and cost-effectiveness analysis, decisions are not based entirely on these measures.

Cost-benefit analysis assigns a dollar value to all costs and benefits of a chosen project. Comparison of the costs and benefits can be used to determine whether a project is worth undertaking. However, the decision to begin or abort further planning may not be based on any cost-benefit analysis.

The formal technique of cost-benefit analysis was introduced by the Corps of Engineers as they began improving U.S. waterways and became mandatory in the Flood Control Act of 1936. Projects initiated under this act required a measure of expected benefits greater than anticipated costs.

During the early 1960s, a cost-benefit approach to decision making was initially adopted by the Department of Defense and later by other governmental agencies. The practice, however, was modified so that most decisions were based on cost effectiveness; that is, once a project was identified as necessary, the process or method to implement it was determined. No serious effort was made to measure the benefits but merely to find the least expensive method to implement the project.

The Federal government eventually adopted a system that combined both cost-benefit and cost-effectiveness analysis for long-range planning and evaluation of existing programs. Even though the system, known as PPBS (Planning-Programming-Budgeting System) was not widely used, it forced government to be more concerned with spending decisions.*

Some problems are inherent to decision making in the public arena. One, which has been brought to our attention recently, is the limited resources of government. Demand for these resources has always exceeded supply. In the past, demand pressures have been substantial because society viewed their needs as a necessary and justifiable means to solve a problem. These demands have not been without merit, and due to political attitudes, commitments for the expenditure of government funds were made. The legal and moral obligations created by these decisions caused government to justify their seeking to increase taxes or increase the

---

*Basic Economic Concepts, Sichet & Eckstain, *Cost Benefit Analysis*, P 337 Rand McNally, 1974

money supply. Today, we are faced with the reality that the bottom of the well may have been reached. Because of this, medical technology research results will become increasingly important in the decision-making arena, particularly if they are cost effective in providing alternatives to current health care practices. Cost-benefit analysis and cost-effectiveness studies will play a more important role in determining payment for new drugs, durable medical equipment, techniques for treating a condition or disease, and even alternative payment methods. An innovation that does not fit the definition of medically necessary in its strictest sense will be eliminated through cost-benefit analysis. These techniques have been used in the past but not pursued as vigorously as we will see in the future.

Research results will become increasingly important. Their impact and use in decision making should be discussed so that there will be common understanding among all parties involved. To begin this process, this paper will address four areas:

1. How medical technology is used in decision making at the state level.
2. Some of the problems, constraints, and barriers faced when establishing policy.
3. How research results are and may be used to aid decision makers.
4. Implications of Federal policies.

BACKGROUND

It must be recognized that Federal and state governments are partners in providing medical care for the categorically needy, ie, poor, disabled, blind, families with dependent children, and aged. Within this partnership, the Federal government issues guidelines that the states must follow. However, a certain amount of leeway is allowed for decision making at the state level where the program is administered.

Each state must have a state plan that describes the benefits the state has agreed to offer. Additionally, any limitation of benefits, method of payment, provision of service procedures, and quality assurance standards must be specified in the state plan. In a sense this document is the contract between state and Federal governments.

Medicaid [Title XIX] and Medicare [Title XVIII] were created in 1965 as amendments to the Social Security Act. The battle to pass these programs was prolonged and emotional because of the involvement of many vested interest groups. Medicare, which was designed to provide medical care for the elderly, took the shape of an insurance program to be administered by the Federal government. Medicaid was established to provide health care for the blind, disabled, aged, and families with dependent children. The amendments required states to provide a portion of the funding for Medicaid and to follow Federal guidelines developed by the Department of Health and Human Services. A mandatory set of services included physician services, lab and x-ray services, in-patient hospital, out-patient hospital, skilled nursing home care, and later family planning, home health, rural health clinics, and EPSDT (Early Periodic Screening, Diagnosis and Treatment) for children under 21 years of age. Other services states wanted to provide were allowed as options. Optional services might include prescription drugs, durable medical equipment, and additional adult services such as eye and dental care. However, these optional services could be subject to certain limitations, such as co-payment.

Creation of a state Medicaid program required enabling state legislation and funding. The form each program took depended upon many forces, including the strength and orientation of lobbying groups, the liberal or conservative bent of legislators, moral issues, and the trust legislators placed in the state agency. As a result, no two states have the same Medicaid program.

Legislative bodies occasionally become a battleground over current Medicaid programs when disagreements arise with administrators. This occurred in Oregon and recently in California, when program administrators created strict closed drug formularies. Legislators in both states responded to pressure groups, including health professionals, manufacturers, and recipients, by introducing legislation that would open the formularies and provide wider coverage. Oregon's legislation passed in 1978 and California's is currently being considered.

The enabling legislation gave administrators of state programs wide latitude in decision making by allowing a certain amount of change within the adopted services. Each state had to adopt a set of regulations to administer the Medicaid program within the definition of the state's enabling legislation. For example, Federal legislation allowed drugs as an optional benefit. If a state's enabling legislation listed prescription drugs as a benefit without limitation, then the administrators had to determine how drugs would be provided, what quantity constraints would apply, how the drugs would be billed to the state, what formula would be used for payment, and which drugs would be offered as a benefit. Drug benefits seem to be one of the controversial areas in most programs. Some states use prior authorization as a utilization control for restricting certain drugs for given uses, such as administering dextroamphetamine for hyperactivity in children and for narcolepsy but not for weight control, or using expensive vitamin preparations (such as Rocaltrol®) for renal dialysis patients. Other states may not pay for certain categories of drugs. Still others may pay for anything a physician orders.

These regulations must conform to Federal requirements, which are published in the Code of Federal Regulations (CFR). This is written by Federal administrators to reflect Title XIX of the Social Security Act and any legislation passed by Congress thereafter. When the Department of Health and Human Services changes its regulations, the states must also change to avoid conflict. If conflict arises, the Federal government can recover the portion of its funds that any state used to pay for a service that did not follow the CFR.

State administrators and legislators are not in complete control of the programs for which they are responsible. The services provided as benefits and reimbursement levels can be set by the government but recipients and health care providers, especially physicians, determine how much of each service is used. Pressure for changes and additions to a program come from this area. Cooperation between government and health care provider groups is especially important for the success of the program.

Government decisions that affect quality of care, benefit changes, or have a fiscal impact must be reviewed and approved by a selected committee and face close scrutiny during funding hearings before state legislative bodies. Administrators who fail to justify their suggestions or actions may not implement their initiative or may have to rescind it if it has been implemented. These programmatic changes must be made through the regulatory process. The decision-making process that leads to program changes is one area where results of medical technology research results become important factors.

Administrators are given a certain level of funding to provide health care for the covered population and are charged with administering their program within that appropriated amount. Furthermore, they are dealing with new technology and ideas that must be evaluated for cost effectiveness. If a new technique or item can be shown to lower the program's costs and maintain the quality of care, the administrator will probably add it as a benefit. This may take the form of adding a new drug to the formulary, paying for a new piece of durable medical equipment, or adding a new procedure code. If the proposed addition does not fit the regulations, however, a change must be made. The change will be researched and written in standard form to be presented, explained, and defended to a select body. In Colorado, this body is the Colorado Board of Social Services, a group created by law to oversee the Department of Social Services programs and whose members are appointed by the Governor.

An example of an added benefit that does not need regulatory changes and appears to be cost effective is the provision of dextrometers for use by diabetic patients. Often a diabetic's blood sugar cannot be measured effectively by urine testing but can be stabilized by using a dextrometer to test blood samples so that insulin can be properly administered. If such a patient can be kept out of the hospital for 2 days, then the cost of the dextrometer is approximately equal to the hospital savings. Thereafter, any reduction in hospital days due to the dextrometer is a savings to the program.

Examples of new concepts that need regulatory or legislative changes are providing health care in alternative settings to delay admissions to nursing homes or adding pharmacy counseling as a reimbursable benefit. The cost effectiveness of each change would have to be considered before regulatory changes would be proposed.

Health care policies are not formulated utilizing cost effectiveness or cost benefit in the purest sense. Moral and emotional issues enter into the decision-making process. For example, End Stage Renal Dialysis (ESRD) is not cost effective but involves emotional issues which include the fear of death and desire to alleviate suffering and pain. Originally, it was felt that offering ESRD would offer some benefit because it would allow patients to return to productive activity. This has not always been the case because the dialyzing process depletes so many chemicals from the patient's body that he or she has little or no strength to participate in former activities. For many, dialysis merely prolongs a painful life. Dialysis treatments can cost approximately $150 three times a week. In addition, the number of drugs needed to cleanse unwanted and potentially dangerous chemicals out of the body, replace vitamins and minerals, and absolve pain are numerous and expensive.

Other similar situations are payment of extensive support, such as hyperalimentation for terminally ill patients; intensive care units for very low birthweight babies whose prognosis for an active, productive life is poor, and heroic efforts to prolong the lives of severe hydro- or microcephalics in public institutions. The decisions to continue this type of care are based purely upon emotional and moral issues that surround the choice between life and death.

Intensive care settings are not the only areas where expenditure and administrative decisions are not based on cost effectiveness. The decision to use government funds to pay only for abortions for the poor when the mother's life is in danger was based upon moral issues. The costs to raise additional children can be prohibitive to welfare recipients who are denied access to abortions because of costs they cannot afford; this is not true for the rest of the population. Therefore, there are two standards of health care in this area—a very prohibitive one for the welfare recipient and a totally accessible one for the patient who can pay the cost of abortion.

Under Medicaid, sterilizations cannot be funded unless an extensive timing schedule and paper trail are followed; such procedures are not required in the private sector. This activity is again the result of moral issues and the Federal government's reaction to an emotional situation.

Cost effectiveness of drugs in the Medicaid program has not been formally measured although all states which include drugs as a benefit assume they are cost effective. Each state has its own method of controlling drug program costs.

It is becoming increasingly clear that the cost effectiveness of some decisions in one area of a program such as pharmacy can be reflected in another portion such as hospitals. The ability to shift funds from one service item to another in those states where budgets are appropriated by line item is becoming increasingly important and necessary. Providing care through home health agencies, providing newer drugs and more durable medical equipment, and realigning certain payment levels to provide better services in a less expensive setting such as the physician's office will thus decrease hospital, nursing home, and out-patient costs. To illustrate that drug costs can be cost effective and decrease expenditures in other areas, a study of the pneumonia vaccination program was initiated during 1978 for Medicaid nursing home patients in Colorado. No formal cost benefit was undertaken to support the program before it was implemented. However, an informal study indicated that a high number of oral cephalosporin prescriptions were being used by nursing home patients for respiratory illnesses, particularly pneumonia. It was felt that five patients could be immunized for the cost of one antibiotic

prescription. When the immunization program was analyzed, surprising results showed that the most significant savings were in in-patient hospital costs. For every $1 spent for the vaccine, $18 in other health costs were saved. In the drug program, $1.95 was saved for every $1 spent. The savings to Medicare were not measured but were probably substantial because Medicare covered in-hospital care for most people in the study group.

A variety of stimuli may trigger an inquiry for change. Some of these come from program staff, health care providers, manufacturers, consumer or recipient groups, legislators, and the courts through their decisions. Once a study area has been identified, the staff formulates the policy change or addition by using a variety of information sources. These can be the results of formal studies, the staffs' own knowledge, court orders, and input from other groups, such as the affected health professionals, recipient groups, or legislators. At this point, medical technology research results become important. The studies must be well written and documented and not appear biased. Merely speculating that a change in a program, such as elimination of certain classes of drugs, will cause an increase in another service, such as hospitalization, is neither helpful nor usable. If no moral or emotional issues are involved, the facts and input are gathered, analyzed, and incorporated into draft regulations to indicate the most cost-effective method of providing the change.

Medical technology research results may not be aimed solely at administrators to be effective. In certain instances it should be offered to others such as legislators. Not only the situations but also the key people who will be most effective in using the research results must be identified.

Changes occur with each set of participants identified. Congressional members can affect national legislation and sometimes administration. Federal and state administrators should be approached if changes in regulations seem appropriate. State legislators deal with specific state problems through their legislative activity. Even lobbying groups can make good use of medical technology research results to effect any change they may want. The identity of the group to approach with information depends on the position of the issue at the time it is being considered. For example, if a new benefit, which has not been previously included in the enabling legislation, is being added to a Medicaid program, then research information should be presented to the legislators and program administrators to support the change. However, if there is any uncertainty about which group or person to approach, the state administrator is generally a good starting point.

PROBLEMS IN ESTABLISHING NEW POLICIES

A variety of problems face administrators when new policies or changes in old ones are proposed. Federal regulations impose barriers that make it difficult to change policies or attempt innovations. The statewide requirement that all services be made available to all recipients in the state restricts tailoring health care services to fit unique sub-population needs. It also precludes testing new concepts in the delivery of health care in one location of the state without obtaining waivers from the Federal government. The waivers involve time and effort to prepare and are difficult to obtain.

Freedom of choice is also a difficult requirement to assure when trying to contain costs or improve services. It requires that recipients be allowed to use any Medicaid qualified provider regardless of cost. This can prevent the state from becoming a prudent purchaser. The only allowable restriction to freedom of choice is lock-in, which allows a state to limit the number of providers overutilizing recipients can use during a given period of time. Recipients who abuse the program can remain eligible for medical assistance if they meet eligibility requirements. States need authority to terminate payment for services to these people.

Co-payments cannot be applied to mandatory services to control usage. A co-payment system could be used to modify the use of some services in certain settings, such as emergency rooms for primary health care. Continuous monitoring of state programs by the Federal government through audits, quality control, state assessments, and validation reviews overlap and tend to tie up state staff whose time is better used to administer the program. Regulations controlling sterilizations, hysterectomies, and abortions are unreasonable and burdensome to both the state and health care providers. This area has cost state programs some good will and cooperation in the health care provider community because of non-payment for services given in good faith but not following exact Federal guidelines.

As Medicaid costs increased, so did the number of Federal regulations. The ability of the state administrators to change their own programs was slowly constricted.

The Reconciliation Act of 1981 began to lift some Federal constraints. Only one section dealt directly with drugs. It requires termination of payment under Medicaid and Medicare Part B for all pre-1962 drugs classified as less than effective as long as a notice for opportunity for hearing has been filed. Elimination of the use of Medicare reasonable charges as an upper limit for Medicaid payment levels for physicians, laboratory services, x-ray, and medical equipment allows states more control over payment levels. Since Medicare is primarily used by the elderly, some procedures used only by a younger population would not have good screens established because of the low number reported. In addition, procedure codes, which differ between Medicare and a state Medicaid program, make translation for the same service and payment level difficult. Now rates can be negotiated with the provider community.

Modification of the freedom of choice provision will allow states to bid competitively for certain services, such as lab and x-ray, if they desire. In addition, recipients can now be required to enroll in a Health Maintenance Organization (HMO) for their health care if one exists in their locality. Waivers will also be given for all services if the state wishes to 1) implement a case management system or specialty physician services arrangement which restricts the provider from whom a recipient can obtain primary health care, 2) use a central broker in a locality, 3) share savings with recipients through added benefits, and 4) institute a lock-in program.

All penalty provisions in the EPSDT program have also been dropped. This allows a state to concentrate on delivery of health care and not the process. Increased coverage under adult day care services through waivers can be obtained if it prevents nursing home admissions. All waivers will be easily obtained. These, in addition to expected changes from the Health Care Financing Administration (HCFA) when regulations are reviewed, will give states a more decisive voice in their own programs.

Other problems facing administrators when program changes are proposed come in the form of pressure group demands. This can be recipient or provider groups as well as other interested citizens. Changes that affect a provider group's payment or participation level, even though it means either less expense for the state or better care for the recipients, may meet resistance. Moves to limit or restrict benefits can face opposition from many directions.

Information is lacking in some areas that could be used to formulate new policies. Innovative reimbursement plans must be designed and studied. Very little research seems to have been done in this area. Models such as those projected by HMOs are used frequently in an attempt to alter other payment mechanisms.

Not only is the lack of information a problem but also the presence of poor information and suspect research results can make change difficult to evaluate or implement.

Policy changes can meet resistance within the organization if jobs or power bases are threatened. If the threat is great enough, the change may fail or not be implemented because of the lobbying efforts of threatened employees.

NEED FOR COST STUDIES

The real need for good research results that provide believable results for decision making is obvious. With funding for public programs becoming tighter, the need to make changes becomes increasingly important. Cost-effectiveness studies resulting in less expensive health care services will be favorably received. Administrators are more likely to respond to a well documented substitution of a less costly service than elimination of a benefit entirely. For example, the use of cimetidine for the treatment of peptic ulcer disease should be presented as cost saving by decreasing the amount of hospitalization and number of operations used previously to treat the condition. A mere statement that this will occur is not enough. Statistics and studies done during the pre-marketing period or information from other areas should be used. However, the cost of misuse should not be neglected when discussing the savings through the use of this or any other product. It becomes harder to justify the continued addition of cephalosporins to Medicaid programs when studies cannot show significant superiority over less costly antibiotics.

An example of a non-drug addition as a benefit would be payment for certain surgical procedures on an out-patient basis only. This substitutes a less costly setting (ie, clinic, physician's office, or out-patient surgical unit) for a more costly one (in-patient hospital).

Research results can be either the primary or secondary basis for the impetus for change. A research article can trigger an administrator's interest to apply the results to his own program. The same article may be used by another administrator to either finish an evaluation or to use it as supporting documentation for proposed changes.

Many research articles do not meet program needs for several reasons. One problem in the pharmaceutical area is the results of a study supplied by company representatives that lists no authors, references, or even source companies. The information is immediately suspect. Even appropriately executed studies are written in such a fashion that they are either hard to understand, present information in a manner not applicable to a public assistance program, or seem to present slanted information.

The source of articles seems to be varied. In addition to articles carried around or relied upon by a vendor or manufacturer's representative to establish a point that appears to enhance his position, research briefs, articles in journals, Federal publications, and conference contacts all are sources of information, which can create interest in a subject leading to further research by the administrator.

IMPLICATIONS OF NEW FEDERAL POLICIES

New Federal policies will change the Medicaid programs. With loosening of Federal control through modification of regulations, states can better control the shape of their programs and tailor them to meet the needs of their people. Fiscal constraints imposed by budget cuts are also going to force changes in each state's program. Some states will be able to maintain the same level of benefits if they can trim some of the unnecessary services, substitute less costly services, or become more efficient in areas such as third party liability recoveries and controlling fraud and abuse. As cuts continue on a yearly basis, then some service areas may have to be limited or eliminated.

If states are awarded block grants and Medicaid is included, then state legislators will take a more active role in determining the shape of their Medicaid program. In most instances, they will be appropriating the money for each program. They will be influenced not only by program administrators but by pressure groups including health care provider and recipient groups. The most powerful and influential group could receive the largest share of the money. However, decisions for distribution of funds at the local level may be more responsive to the needs of the community. It is hoped that legislators will leave much of the decision making to the administrators or at least rely upon their advice so the integrity of each program will remain intact.

CONCLUSIONS

There is a need for cost-benefit and cost-effectiveness analysis in the health care area. This is particularly true now that fiscal constraints are becoming the driving force behind program designs. Research projects are needed in areas such as less expensive alternatives to present service benefits and innovative reimbursement mechanisms that are cost effective without diminishing the quality of care. Introduction of new goods or services that might be reimbursable under Medicaid must be shown to be cost effective as well as medically necessary before they will be considered as benefits. If the studies are well done, they can be of great benefit to the program administrators and ultimately to the taxpayers as well as the recipients eligible to receive benefits under the Medicaid program.

Discussion

Question: It seems that none of the studies mentioned has been developed in a welfare or Medicaid population. I don't think that the conclusions drawn by some of the studies can be extrapolated to Medicaid patients, who are basically a nonproductive welfare population. The cause of their nonproductivity, and whether cost-benefit analysis using the methods in the current studies can bring any information to bear on the decision-making process in a Medicaid program, is unclear to me. I think we have to go several steps further. A model using that particular population would be useful to Medicaid state administrators.

Response: It is risky to extrapolate data from one population in which a study was conducted to a different population. It is also difficult to make economic projections of the consequences of employability or improved function in a population that is underemployed or unemployed relative to one that is fully employed.

Geweke and Weisbrod studied the impact of cimetidine in a Medicaid population in Texas. After controlling for severity of disease and other features, the best prediction they were able to make from the evidence was that the drug did introduce a net cost savings in the medical care of those patients. One might ask what the Medicaid population in Texas has to do with the Medicaid population in New Jersey, one can get into an infinite series of questions as to whether a study of one population applies to another. Physicians can also ask how one study relates to an individual patient.

We have a tendency at times to concentrate on cost savings to measure worth. We use a term like cost effectiveness when we are actually talking about net dollar savings for a specific program or state. Depending on the point of view of a particular agency, the net cost consequences of an innovation like cimetidine can be negative or positive. For example, antacids are not currently covered in Louisiana's Medicaid program. But in Pennsylvania and many other states, many over-the-counter drugs, including antacids, are covered. It may well be that the amount of antacids taken is reduced when patients also take cimetidine. To someone responsible for the pharmacy budget in a state Medicaid program already paying for antacids, it may look as though the state is paying more for cimetidine, but realizing other compensating savings. If antacids aren't covered, the state's pharmacy budget will not reflect those savings.

An extension of that is the point Dr. Myers made in her discussion of the pneumococcal vaccine. The Medicaid budget experienced substantial savings, but she commented that the Medicare program experienced even greater savings. I think we should be wary of thinking that our own budgets represent or reflect what is socially useful. Neither Medicare nor Medicaid has anything to do with employment and the indirect economic benefits of interventions that allow people to return to work. There may be net cost savings to society that transcend any one budget.

Weighing benefits against net costs, when there are no net savings, presents a difficult problem. To what extent should we support those innovations, interventions, or technologies that cost money, but that also provide health benefits?

Response: Unfortunately, California is faced with a problem related to size and the length of time it takes to do a cost-benefit or cost-effectiveness analysis in order to help make any decision. The emotion tied to the decision-making process comes through different routes—the legislature, the necessity for fast action, and the provider groups that may be affected by the resulting decision. If we had the luxury and the ability to take the risk of going the cost-benefit route, we would probably end up with the kind of decision that would be the most intelligent, but not necessarily the most expedient for the particular condition at that time. California's Medicaid budget, which is a significant portion of the state's overall budget and deficit, is the largest single state program consuming about 12.5% of the state's budget. Consequently trade-offs and decisions must be made somewhere. In that type of situation, you don't have the luxury of deciding what is most cost effective or has the greatest cost benefit. It boils down to a more pragmatic kind of decision-making process, which must be made in the face of many constraints. At the staff level, many times cost-benefit analyses have already been done and the results come to the decision makers in the form of a recommendation in which choices are laid out on a rational basis. However, when the decision has to be made, it may be reached from an irrational, illogical basis.

Response: The extreme pressure and distress facing Medicaid programs across the country today are really not appreciated. Medicaid is also the largest single program in Michigan, as it is in about two thirds of the states. Last year Michigan actually experienced a $300 million decline in state revenues. Nevertheless, in that year the Medicaid program expanded by $160 million, meaning that the state government had to absorb nearly $500 million. There is pressure on all departments to decrease spending and budgets are being cut drastically while at the same time payments to physicians, hospitals, and pharmacists are going up. In this context it is unreasonable to talk about applying cost-benefit analysis where the criterion is coverage of a particular product or drug that will offer benefit, because we are talking about eliminating drugs or items within Medicaid coverage that are less effective than those that would remain. This is extremely distressing to me personally. In Michigan we have always operated the Medicaid program on the premise that we would pay for whatever the physician determined medically necessary. Unlike many other states we have had few restrictions on drugs, hospital coverage, physician visits, and the like. But economic necessity has forced us away from this principle. In the last 2 weeks we have had to eliminate coverage for drugs such as antacids, laxatives, cough and cold preparations, vitamins, and others. These are very difficult decisions that have therapeutic consequences.

Other examples fall outside the drug arena. On the first of January we terminate coverage for some 28 inpatient surgical procedures that can be performed on an outpatient basis. Hereafter, we will only cover these as outpatient procedures. These decisions are being made with imperfect information. Cost-benefit or cost-effectiveness analysis provides one vehicle for bringing that information to the decision makers, but the information is not free. All information costs, and somebody has to pay that cost; often no one is willing to pay the cost. So we make decisions using whatever information we have available and hope for the best.

Response: We must not lose sight of the fact that the purpose of health care is not to save money, but to provide health. One aspect or underlying principle of cost-effectiveness analysis is distinct from cost-benefit analysis. The supposition in cost-effectiveness analysis is that resources are limited and that the objective is to provide as much health care as possible. Then it seems clear that it is too stringent a test to require that any new procedure save money. If it buys health in a reasonable way compared with other potential uses of those resources, then perhaps it ought to be undertaken and covered under state Medicaid and federal Medicare programs.

What troubles me, though, is an asymmetry between the stringency of the test applied to new procedures and technologies and the stringency of the test applied to existing procedures and technologies. Five or 10 years ago, health economists and various critics of the health care system selected from an economic point of view three potentially explosive technologies— coronary bypass surgery, CT scanning, and cimetidine—that they feared would result in widespread application of inefficacious medicine. As it has turned out, numerous studies including efficacy studies, cost-effectiveness studies, and others indicate that when appropriately used these are all extremely cost effective. On the other hand, a number of widely used existing procedures clearly do not save money, for example, hysterectomies for fibroid tumors. Analysis has shown that they are not very cost effective.

Response: It seems clear that states traditionally operate on a crisis intervention basis, which we cannot avoid because we work with taxpayers' money. And as the economy changes, the available resources change. But one thing that has become clear is that there are parallel courses. Even though we may have to take the crisis intervention route at any given point, that doesn't preclude taking the parallel course of using cost-benefit and cost-effectiveness analyses for long-term planning and evaluation and, in the process, reevaluate what we have done during the crisis. In the case of Michigan removing some drugs from their formulary, I would want to evaluate the effects of that particular action in light of this symposium.

Priorities for Future CBA/CEA in Policymaking

Paul D. Stolley, M.D.

Professor of Medicine and Co-Director of the Clinical Epidemiology Unit
Section of General Medicine
Department of Medicine
University of Pennsylvania School of Medicine
Philadelphia, Pennsylvania

INTRODUCTION

Simply stated, cost-benefit analysis is an evaluation of the money you spend or sacrifice in relation to the value, again in terms of money, of what you get. It is a systematic approach to decision making that should be the economic basis on which choices and trade-offs are made. As applied to the health care system, cost-benefit analysis considers the costs of medical care in respect to the loss of net earnings due to death or disability. If the monetarized benefits of medical care exceed its costs, then that particular use of resources appears to make economic sense, although not as much sense as some other use, resulting in benefits exceeding the costs even more. This principle holds for *all* economic decisions.

Medical care over the past 2 decades has been characterized by rapid technological development. If we think about pacemakers, computerized axial tomography (CAT), coronary bypass procedures, renal dialysis, insulin infusion pumps, and the application of genetic engineering to the manufacture of biologicals and pharmaceuticals, we can begin to appreciate the impact of the technological revolution on health care services.

In the coming decade we will undoubtedly witness an explosion in the introduction of new technology in medical care. Some of the areas marked for future development are: noninvasive high-resolution imaging such as the PET scan; application of genetic engineering to the production of new pharmaceuticals and hormones (such as human growth hormone and interferon); improvement of new prosthetic devices; and computerization of record keeping and other aspects of patient care and practice management. In the area of pharmaceuticals, it is expected that important drugs will be introduced into the market for the prevention of myocardial infarction, the treatment and prevention of peptic ulcer disease and possibly vaccines for certain cancers such as hepatic cancer, Burkitt's Lymphoma or cervical cancer.

IMPORTANCE OF EVALUATION STUDIES

Epidemiologists have long stressed the importance of properly evaluating the efficacy of these new therapies and technologies by experimental methods. It is noteworthy that coronary artery bypass graft was not subjected to study by randomized controlled trials until about 50,000 bypass procedures were being performed annually in the United States. Even now this procedure is being performed for indications for which there has been no proof of efficacy. Similarly, CAT scanners were purchased before anyone had analyzed their cost in relation to alternative diagnostic methods.

The theoretical rationale behind experimental designs to evaluate new technology was described by Sir R.A. Fisher[1] in the early 1930s and popularized to the medical community by Sir Austin Bradford Hill several years later. Because methods of evaluating new therapies and technologies are highly developed, there is scant intellectual excuse for not performing appropriate randomized controlled trials. Several reasons have been offered to explain this reluctance to apply the experimental method: ignorance, adherence to tradition, and a rush to cash in on commercial investments, to name a few.

It is necessary to conduct randomized controlled trials to evaluate efficacy because cost-benefit and cost-effectiveness analyses are impossible without a reliable estimate of the medical benefit of a new procedure. At the present time the randomized controlled trial is the most powerful and reliable means of assessing benefit. Often the benefits of a new procedure are not adequately assessed. Such was the case with the Papanicolaou cytology technique for the early diagnosis of cervical carcinoma. Before the value of this procedure was demonstrated, the twice-yearly "Pap smear" had become a routine component of women's health care. Only recently has the Pap smear's impact on reducing morbidity and mortality from this tumor been shown. The time interval between Pap smears, as well as the ages at which it should be performed, are still under review. Meanwhile, an entire "Pap smear industry" was created, and any controlled trial to test the efficacy of this screening technique would be virtually impossible because of the premature advocacy of this method by practitioners and pathologists.

CRITICISMS OF COST-BENEFIT ANALYSIS

One would think that such a systemic approach to decision making as cost-benefit analysis would be generally supported and relatively noncontroversial. However, this is not the case. The rationale for cost-benefit analysis, as well as its underlying moral philosophy, have been sharply questioned by some opponents.

One of the major criticisms levied against cost-benefit analysis is that it attempts to make decisions in situations where cost cannot be quantified, or where reasonable persons would disagree about *how* to calculate the costs and their *extent*. How, for example, *does* one quantify human suffering, grief, or the ravages of disease, or even war for that matter? The difficulty of quantifying such qualities is well-illustrated in this quotation from the famous radio play entitled "On A Note of Triumph" by Norman Corwin. It was written in 1945 in preparation for victory in Europe and broadcast on the day that the victory over the fascists was announced. The play attempted to help the American public understand the causes and costs of World War II. In discussing the costs of the war, the narrator says:
The deep red gouge across the inner calculations is the trail of hate,
and there is no accounting for the turns it will take, both sooner and later.
The slide rule, faced with this, is panicky and sterile, and algebra goes home to die among the Arabs.
Shall the balance sheet be balanced? By whom? How?
No combination of savants and learned cogs, holes punched in cards and electric motors,
No brow containing Euclid, not even the serenest lores in consultation with each other
could be else than baffled by the simplest problem of the cost of hunger in a baby's bones.
And if you wish to assess the cost of beating the fascists, you must multiply the number of closed files in the departments of war, by the exchange value of sorrow,
which is infinite and has no decimals.[2]

The critics of cost-benefit analysis reject the notion that a universal measure of cost can be, or even should be, quantified in terms of dollars or some other economic unit. They might cite, as an example of their philosophic stance, the premature death of a mother "on welfare," pointing out that if her lost earnings were computed they would amount to nothing, and that, in fact, she and her children were supported by the State. Therefore, in the context of a cost-benefit analysis framework, any disease she would experience would have little "cost" attached to it (assuming that the emotional and social cost of the loss of a mother to her children is not entered into such simple calculations). Applying this kind of "straw man" model to another example, suppose a wealthy executive of a cigarette manufacturing company were to sustain a premature death. In this case, there would be a large loss of future earnings despite the fact that this work was detrimental to society.

Another general criticism of cost-benefit analysis is that it can be extremely imprecise, and consequently easily manipulated and misused in order to defend a particular viewpoint. A recent illustration of this problem is provided by the controversy over the costs of various regulatory agencies and government regulations designed to protect workers at the workplace or to protect citizens from pollution by industry. Murray Weidenbaum, while an economist at the Center for the Study of American Business, calculated that in 1979 the Government spent $5.8 billion to run all of its regulatory agencies, and that businesses spent $116 billion to comply with the regulations of these agencies. These estimates have been contested by other economists, such as William Tabb, who maintained that a more realistic estimate of all regulatory costs would be $54 billion, or less than half of the figure computed by Weidenbaum.[3]

Another controversial example is a cost-benefit analysis conducted by Sam Peltzman, an economist who worked with Milton Friedman's group in Chicago. Dr. Peltzman tried to assess the costs of the 1962 Kefauver legislation. This Act tightened up safety procedures for the marketing of drugs and required that the efficacy of new drugs be demonstrated (usually with controlled clinical trials) prior to marketing. He concluded that the costs of these regulations outweighed their benefits, but his calculations of costs and benefits have been challenged.[4]

A new attack has been launched on cost-benefit analysis by labor union economists and "consumer protection" groups who perceive the technique as both crude and primarily serving the political and economic interests of business and management.

In medical care, the use of cost-benefit analysis is confounded in much the same manner as it is in other fields. This conceptually simple and presumably equitable approach can be quite difficult to implement. For example, if one were analyzing the costs of air pollution, some of the costs could be easily assessed—extra laundry or house-painting bills incurred as a direct result of air pollution from a nearby factory. Others would be more difficult. As Willian Ophuls stated: "most of the costs cannot be readily quantified—for example, the health effects of air pollution, for it is almost impossible to know who suffers, to what degree, from what amount, of which agents. Besides, what is the economic cost of a life? A reduced life span? The risk of contracting emphysema? Being forced by smog to stay inside?"[5]

In the case of air pollution, it is difficult to determine *who* sustains the cost and *what* are the actual damages to health. It may be years before we understand the damages specifically attributable to air pollution. Given that some of the costs attributable to air pollution are unknown at the present time, we might perform a cost-benefit analysis which seriously *under*estimated or *over*estimated costs. Cost-benefit analysis is, therefore, of little help when one is ignorant of either costs or benefits; it can sometimes give the impression that there is greater knowledge than is actually the case.

FUTURE APPLICATIONS OF COST-BENEFIT ANALYSIS IN MEDICAL CARE

Economists, in collaboration with medical care researchers and practitioners, are beginning to apply cost-benefit and cost-effectiveness analyses for the evaluation and assessment of new therapies and new technologies. Cimetidine, for example, has been the object of just such intense study; the benefits of the drug have been measured not only in terms of the avoidance of morbidity and mortality using disability days, lost earnings, avoidance of premature death and hospitalization costs, but there has also been an attempt to determine if the introduction of this drug has affected rates of surgical procedures for intractable peptic ulcer and other complications requiring operation. Recent work published by Dr. Harvey Fineberg showed a decrease in gastric operations usually associated with peptic ulcer disease at about the time cimetidine was introduced.[6] It will be interesting to see if a similar decline in surgical procedures occurs in countries that did *not* market cimetidine or in areas where the drug was *not* widely used. Regression techniques can be used to determine whether there is a correlation between cimetidine use and a decrease in surgical procedures. Such observational studies are helpful, but, of course, inferences must be stated cautiously. Whether or not a quasi-experimental or randomized controlled trial could be employed to study new drugs or procedures once marketed, is problematic. Although these research strategies are more powerful than nonexperimental methods, the logistics of sample size, ethics, and costs may prevent their application during the post-marketing period when continued surveillance would be important.

To evaluate properly the fruits of medical technology as they affect the health care sector, greater attempts must be made to delineate the *intangible costs* associated with the introduction of these technologies aimed at diagnosing and treating disease: the pain and discomfort of illness, grief over the death of persons with that illness, and so on. These elusive intangible costs are rarely accounted for because they are so difficult to define and measure.

Cost-effectiveness analysis is an attractive alternative or supplement to cost-benefit analysis. The measurement of effectiveness has been the concern of epidemiologists, statisticians, and economists. Epidemiologists in particular have criticized the assumption often held by health agency officials that programs are effective before being proved effective. Health education programs have often been *assumed* to be effective simply because they intuitively seem so reasonable. When rigorous efforts are made to measure their effectiveness, the programs are sometimes found deficient. An example of this fallacy is illustrated by the attempt to evaluate educational programs designed to increase the use of seat belts in communities. Through the use of television, radio, and newspapers, clever messages were beamed at a target population urging the use of seat belts. Surveys of seat belt use before and after this expensive program showed little change in use—and a small amount of change suggested *decreased* use of seat belts.

Future cost-benefit analysis should focus more sharply on two problems, one method logistically soluble at present, and the other, more intractable. The more tractable problem is that of effectiveness evaluation of health programs prior to cost-benefit analysis. As previously mentioned, controlled clinical trials, quasi-experimental designs such as those used in programs to control coronary heart disease, the seat belt study just cited, and pilot studies can contribute to the measurement of the effectiveness of health programs. A successful example of such an evaluation is the now famous two-city study of the effect of adding fluoride to the city water supply. Measures of diseased, missing, and filled teeth before and after the addition of fluoride to one of the community's water supply showed a clear difference between the two communities.

This result led the late George James to observe that the addition of fluoride by a single uneducated individual shovelling it into the New York City reservoirs did more to affect dental caries than the work of 10,000 expensive and highly educated dentists.

Quasi-experimental designs have helped to evaluate large-scale community programs designed to reduce morbidity and mortality due to coronary heart disease. According to a letter from P. Puska, MD, Head, North Karelia Project, in July, 1980, an ambitious program in the province of North Karelia, Finland, has shown that mortality and morbidity rates attributed to stroke may be reduced by such programs. There is hopeful evidence that the same can be shown for reduction in coronary heart disease as well. In their book *Quasi-Experimentation,* Campbell and Stanley state that the inferential power of the quasi-experimental design chosen tends to be inversely related to its feasibility; yet as a technique it certainly represents an advance over the previous uncontrolled trials commonly used to evaluate health programs.[7]

The *less* tractable problem concerns the measurement of the so-called intangible costs of disease. Here the realms of philosophy, judgment, politics, and ethics come together. An example of the difficulty of measuring intangible costs is illustrated by the argument of some free-market economists that drug regulation may, in the long run, be more costly than an unregulated market. Arthur Okun, commenting on this, said "some situations cry out for public intervention. For example, it is cold comfort that, without food and

drug regulation, a consumer who is fatally poisoned by a medication will never buy that product again."[8] In the example cited by Okun there is clear conflict between the kind of moral outrage a consumer feels when he or she is misled, cheated, or subjected to premature release of an untested therapy, as contrasted to the possible efficiencies and reduced costs industry may enjoy when such regulation is abandoned.

FUTURE TECHNOLOGICAL ADVANCES THAT WILL REQUIRE EVALUATION

The coming decade may see the following advances in medicine:
- Increased laser surgery
- Computer-assisted vision and hearing
- Myoelectronic prosthetic hands where a machine is "directed" by the patient's own muscles, to replace hands accidentally amputated.
- Further development of artificial joints
- Work on artificial blood substitutes
- Introduction of an artificial heart
- Portable renal dialysis machinery
- Manipulation of genes to "instruct" cancerous cells to stop dividing
- Screening tests for early detection of cancers or to identify persons at high risk of cancer
- Use of constant infusion insulin pumps.

These developments are among many which will have to be evaluated; cost-benefit and cost-effectiveness analyses will certainly contribute to this evaluation.

Paradoxically, along with this burgeoning technology is a concomitant decline in public health services. Toxic and nuclear wastes, garbage and industrial and automotive pollutants are not properly disposed of; many of our poor do not have access to medical and dental services, and the elderly ill are badly provided for. The medical profession is still hindered by the "impedimenta" of unevaluated procedures and remedies: complicated machinery for the treatment of chronic respiratory disease, hormonal treatment of the menopause, and tonsillectomies for trivial indications, to mention a few. Although some efficacy studies have been done, as with tonsillectomies and adenoidectomies, a profitable procedure dies slowly. Studying this again is a kind of "intellectual archeology" with little appeal for researchers.

PROBLEMS AND ISSUES

One important practical difficulty encountered in the past (and likely to recur, if measures are not taken to correct it) is the lag between the introduction of medical innovations and the initiation and completion of cost-benefit, cost-effectiveness or other evaluative studies. Coronary artery bypass graft and CAT scans are examples where studies have lagged behind the adoption and widespread use of these procedures. Short of legislative requirements, an economic system that provides incentives for new technology is hard to "slow down" for the critical studies. In England, where the state must purchase new medical technology, these studies are more likely to precede adoption of new technology. If medical insurers (third party payers) were somehow penalized for covering unproven innovations, or if incentives to conduct these studies were somehow provided, they might be encouraged to a greater extent in the United States. The work of the Office of Technology Assessment of the U.S. Congress is certainly an encouraging development.

A current interest in postmarketing medical technology surveillance has both positive and negative aspects, in my opinion. The positive side of this interest is the increased attention paid to the effects—either adverse or beneficial—in populations over the years. The negative side may be the attempt to weaken premarketing testing of drugs and other technology based on the presence of the "safety net" of the postmarketing surveillance system. We still are ignorant about the feasibility, utility, and sensitivity of such a surveillance system, and until we have demonstrated how it works, it may be premature to loosen up premarketing testing requirements.

Of course, the very best test of efficacy (at least the most decisive and convincing) is the randomized controlled trial (RCT). These trials are often large, lengthy, expensive, and difficult to mount. They may involve multiple clinical centers and thus pose formidable logistical problems. Nevertheless, the potential contribution of such RCTs can be enormous. The Coronary Drug Project, University Group Diabetes Project, the VA Trial of Anti-Hypertensive Therapy, and the Multiple Risk Factor Intervention Trial (MRFIT) are examples of large-scale RCT's designed to answer crucial questions of medical care efficacy and effectiveness. However, recent uncontrolled trials of total lymphoid irradiation for intractable rheumatoid arthritis led an editorialist for the *New England Journal of Medicine* to warn that "the genie not be allowed to escape from the bottle again," a reference to the coronary bypass experience.[9] There is still no adequate substitute to RCT's for the answering of many questions.

Summary

Cost-benefit and cost-effectiveness analyses are useful methods, if properly applied, for quantifying and assessing the effects of medical innovations. They aid policy-makers in choosing between options and present data which help organize debate over policy. Like any useful tool, eg, statistical analysis or laboratory tests, the method can be misapplied or deliberately distorted in the service of special interests. When fairly applied, however, these kinds of analyses represent a considerable advance over testimonial, anecdotal or emotionally presented information.

REFERENCES

1. Fisher RA: *Design of Experiments.* London, Oliver & Boyd, 1935
2. Corwin N: *On A Note of Triumph.* New York, Simon and Schuster, 1945
3. Reagonomics: A Dollars and Sense Pamphlet. Economic Affairs Bureau, Somerville, MA, 1981, p 15
4. Peltzman S: An evaluation of consumer protection legislation: the 1962 drug amendments. *Journal of Political Economy* 81(Sept/Oct), 1973
5. Ophuls W: *Ecology and the Politics of Scarcity.* San Francisco, W.H. Freeman and Co, 1977
6. Fineberg HU, Pearlman LA: Center for the Analysis of Health Practices, CHAP News Letter Cimetidine or Surgery for the Treatment of Ulcer, vol. 4, 1981
7. Campbell D, Stanley JC: *Experimental and Quasi-Experimental Designs for Research.* Chicago, Rand McNally, 1966
8. Okun M: *The Political Economy of Prosperity.* The Brookings Institution, Washington, D.C., 1970
9. McCarty DJ: Treating intractable arthritis. *New England Journal of Medicine* 305:1009–1011, 1981

Discussion

PRIORITIES IN SELECTING ISSUES FOR EVALUATION

Comment: There is a completely different way of looking at criteria to determine the best set of candidates for limited evaluation dollars. We might start by focusing on the health care reimbursement and regulatory systems and on the incentives to providers and consumers of health care. Given that system, what technologies are likely to be adopted too rapidly or too slowly or perhaps not at all? In the first category, new procedures that can be developed or performed by physicians and therefore can be brought in at high reimbursement rates under the prevailing system of physician reimbursement might be good candidates for rapid deployment. For instance, endoscopy is paid at very high physician reimbursement rates, which have stayed high as a result of the system of physician reimbursement. Those technologies that are likely to be adopted slowly might include rehabilitation, where the benefits of the technology cannot be captured due to difficulty or a dispersed market. Thus, we might be able to identify technologies that might have the greatest impact on program expenditures and therefore might need evaluation, and we might also be able to identify which Medicaid or public policies, with regard to reimbursement and regulation, are most in need of careful scrutiny.

Dr. Stolley: It has always struck me as curious that physicians are reimbursed at high rates for passing tubes. Yet, if physicians decide to spend 30 minutes with patients to comfort and reassure them and discuss a personal problem, they are hardly reimbursed at all. Clearly, the reimbursement system encourages certain overutilization and underutilization.

Question: We have been dealing with the application of cost-benefit and cost-effectiveness analyses for future technologies. What are the future methodologies that we might use to tackle some of the existing technologies so that policymakers have further tools at their disposal to evaluate more appropriately the costs, effects, benefits, risks, and even the political and social implications of some of their decisions?

Dr. Stolley: Postmarketing surveillance could be used, not just for drugs but for a variety of other procedures. This can be used to pick up unexpected efficacy.

Response: As part of a study that has not as yet been published, we have been trying to extend the use of nonexperimental epidemiologic techniques beyond their usual application, studying adverse drug reactions and drug efficacy in postmarketing surveillance. In general, this has been considered invalid mainly because patients who receive a drug are in some way inherently different from those who do not. A blatant example might be nonexperimentally studying whether propranolol prevented sudden death. You would see more sudden death in people receiving propranolol than in those who have not received the drug. That difference between the treated and the untreated patients, which epidemiologists call confounding by the indication for therapy, has been thought to make nonexperimental studies of drug efficacy impossible. We have been developing methodologies and looking for situations where drug efficacy can best be studied nonexperimentally. These techniques will never be as convincing as experimental trials nor are they intended to replace the randomized clinical trial. Rather, their use is to supplement in situations where randomized clinical trials are either unethical or logistically impossible, or not worth the cost entailed for the question being addressed. Basically, it is possible, in certain circumstances, to study drug efficacy by nonexperimental trials, which is a methodology that I hope will be used more widely in the future.

Dr. Stolley: Two nonexperimental methods have already been introduced. One is the case-control method. For example, elderly women who have sustained fractures can be compared to a control group to find out whether the elderly women who had the fractures took less medication that is thought to prevent fractures, such as estrogen or calcium supplements. Sometimes a clue to efficacy can be obtained by this retrospective or case-control method. The other is a cohort method. Using the same example, one might evaluate a group of women taking estrogen to control certain symptoms of the menopause to see if they have fewer fractures as time progresses than women who don't use estrogen. These nonexperimental designs create problems, and one must be cautious about inferences.

Response: Some other techniques coming into greater use have been used in other fields. Randomized trials, or even the quasi-experimental trials, tend to focus on before-and-after events. Yet Markovian and semi-Markovian processes can be adapted to look at changes through the entire process of the intervention procedures and to evaluate them in both a process format and a final outcome format. New ideas and new applications of methodology in that area should start opening up in the medical field. It is being used somewhat in certain areas, but not nearly enough in other areas. People undergoing some kind of intervention go through changes in either their health status or economic status. Looking at those changes and how they influence future paths and future decisions through the intervention phase can be a fruitful area of research and therefore lead to better cost-effectiveness and cost-benefit analyses.

Response: Another perspective on the problem is that we are trying to optimize something within various resource constraints—personnel, funding availability, and things of that sort. In the abstract that sounds like a linear or mathematical programming problem. Instead of looking at something that seeks to maximize national income, which is essentially a cost-benefit computation, maybe we have to look at optimization within constraints that also gets us out of the internal rate of return bind.

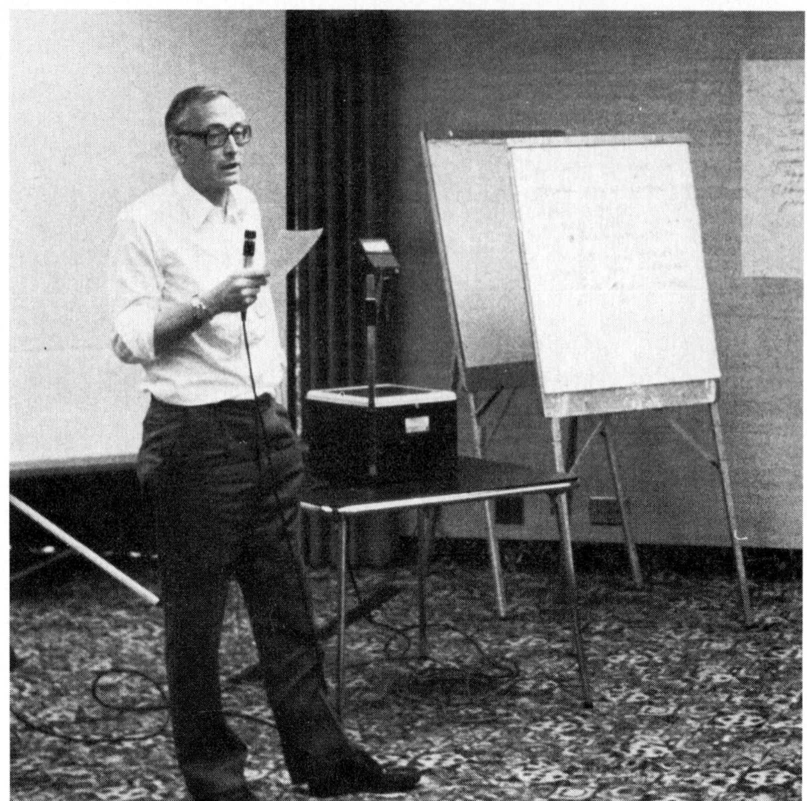
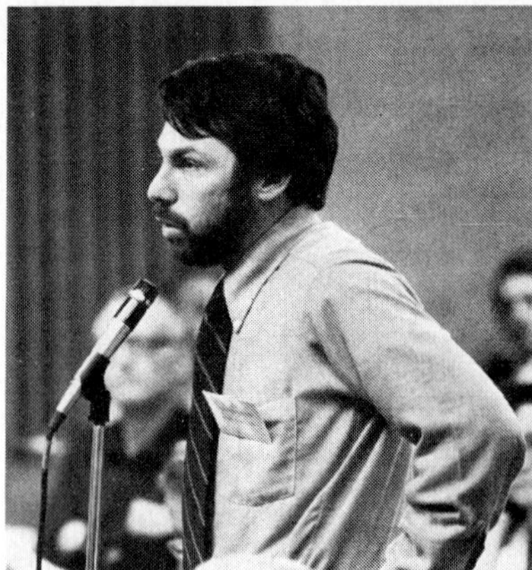

Sandford J. Schwartz, M.D.

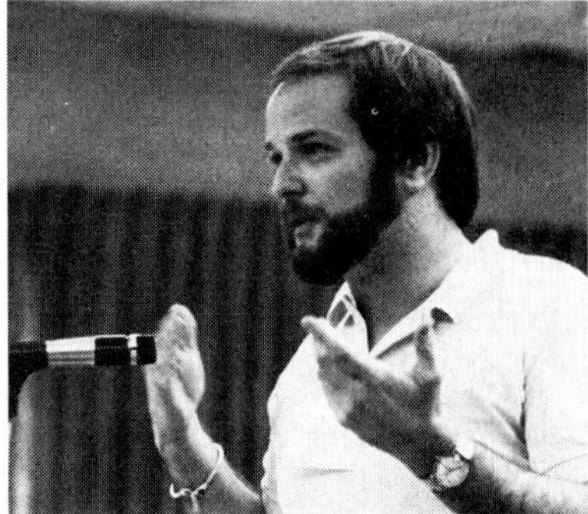

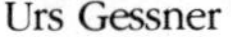

Urs Gessner

Harry M. Rosen, Ph.D.

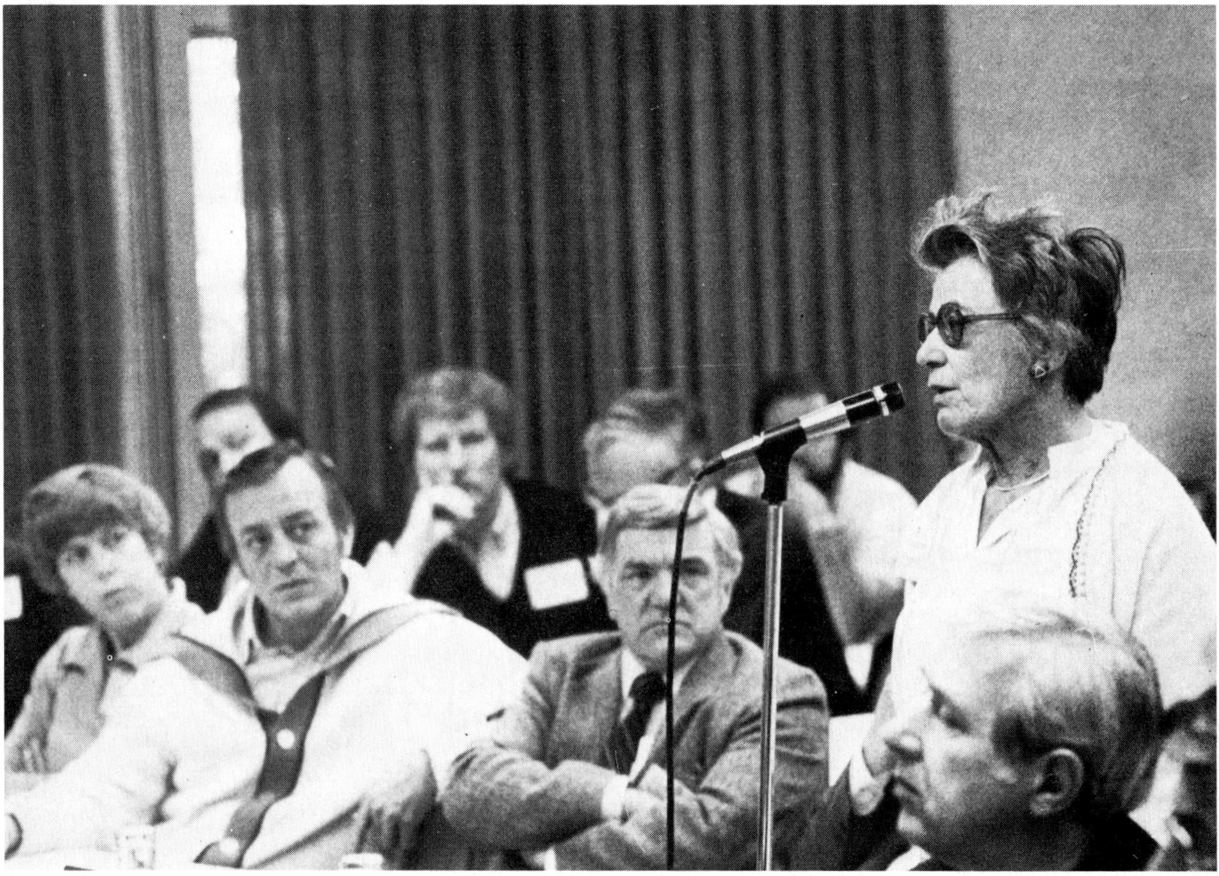

Rita Ricardo-Campbell, Ph.D.; (l-r) Myrle A. Myers, R.Ph.; Arthur E. Cocco, M.D.; Michael P. O'Donnell, R.Ph ; Louis Kolek, R.Ph.

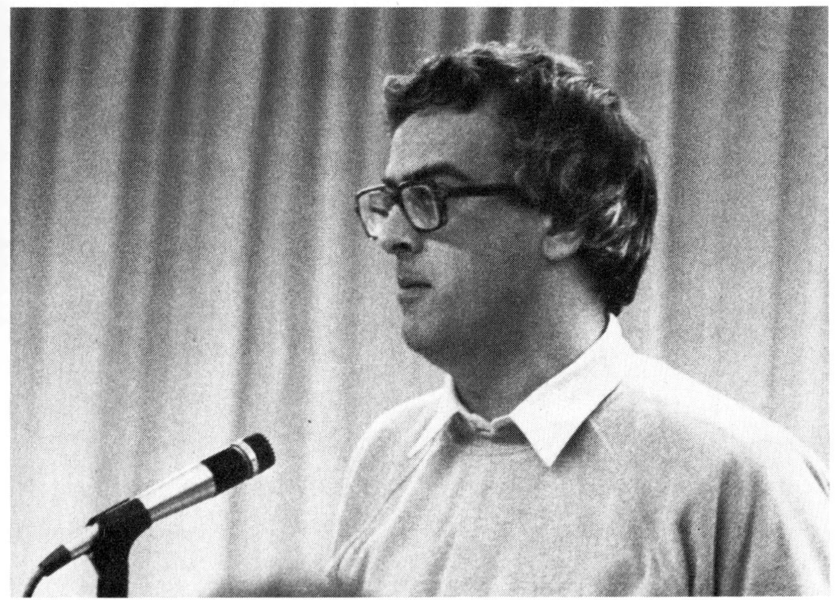

Anthony J. Culyer, Ph.D.

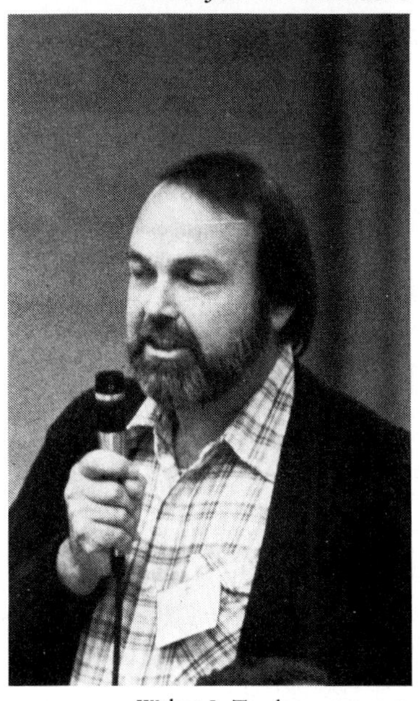

Walter L Trudeau, B.M. B.Ch.

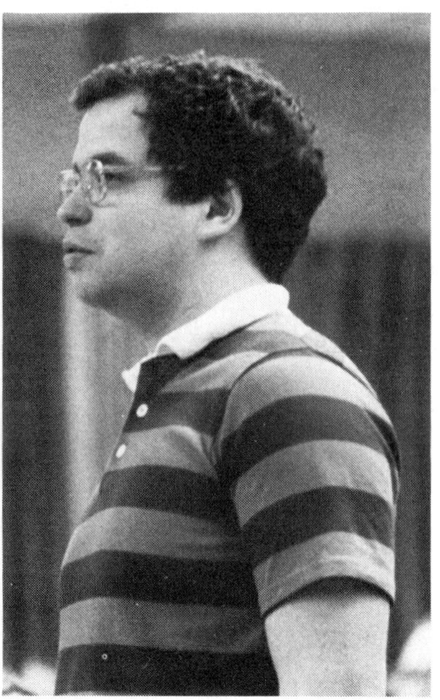

Milton C. Weinstein, Ph.D.

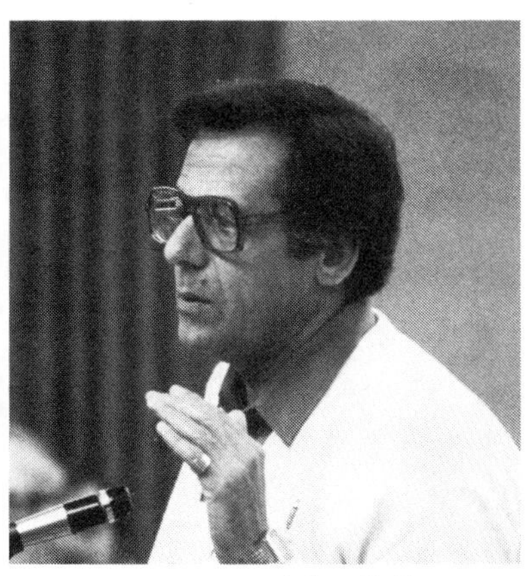

Arthur E. Cocco, M.D.

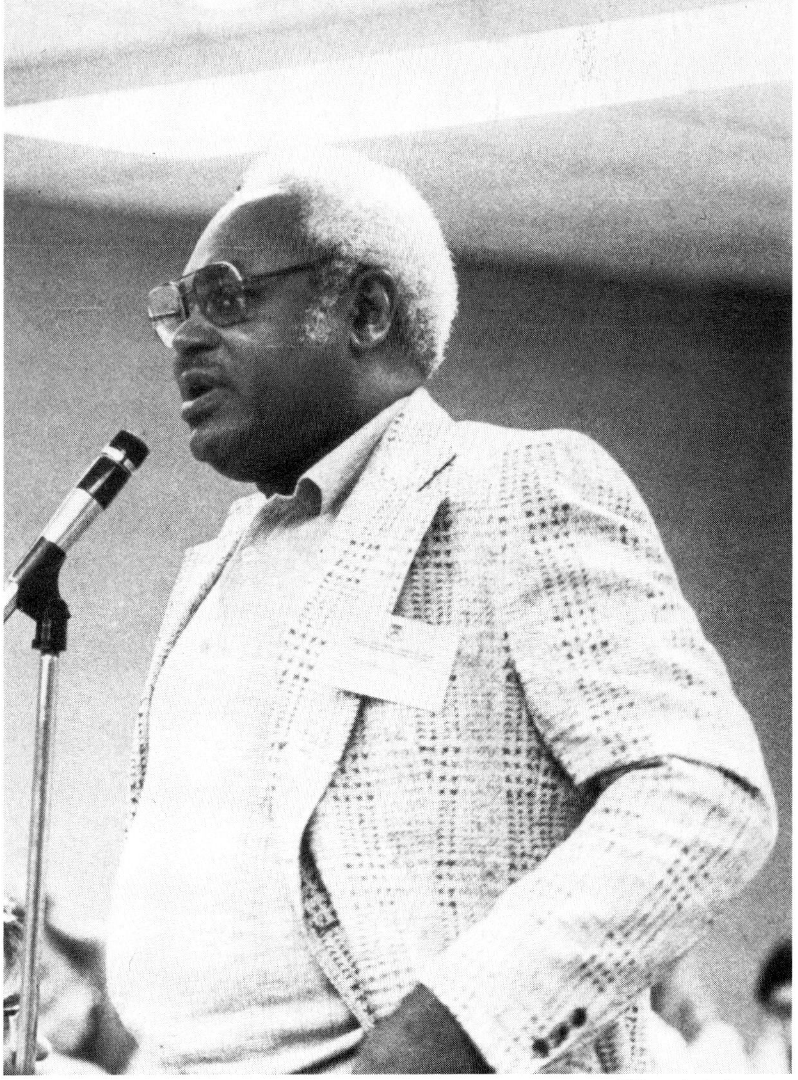

Clifton A. Cole, M.P.A.

CHAPTER III

Consensus of Working Group Sessions

Theme I:
Use of CBA/CEA in Policymaking
Harvey V. Fineberg, M.D., Ph.D.

Theme II:
Integration of Research Results with External Factors in the Policy and Decision-Making Process
James T. Doluisio, Ph.D.

Theme III:
Priorities for Future Studies of Medical Technology
Clifton A. Cole, M.P.A.

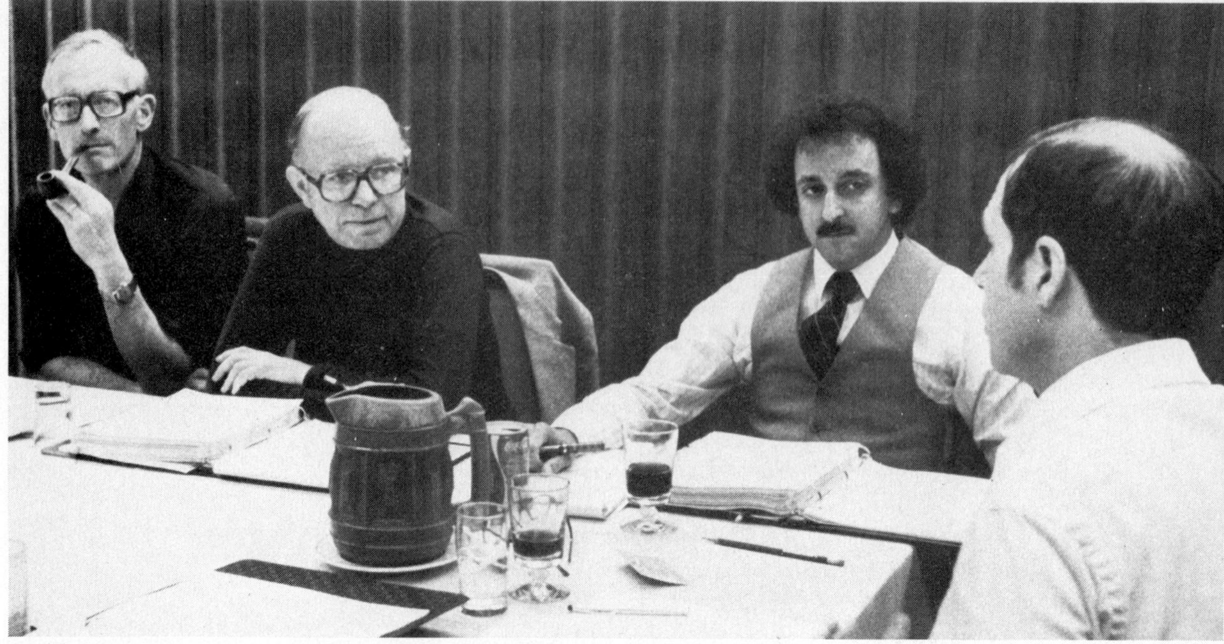

(l-r) Urs Gessner; Robert C. Jones, Ph.D. Joseph E. Concino, R.Ph. Paul D. Stolley, M.D., M.Ph.

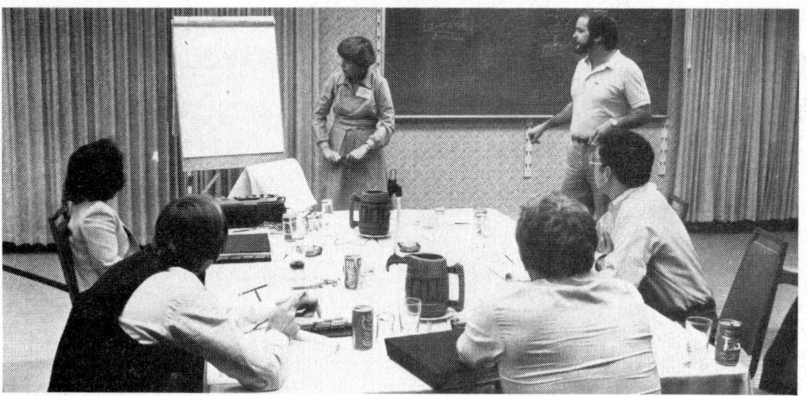

(l-r) Thi D. Dao, Ph.D. Vernon K. Smith, Ph.D.; Myrle A. Myers, R.Ph.; The Honorable Tarkey
J. Lombardi, Jr.; John A. Pagliarini; Harry M. Rosen, Ph.D.

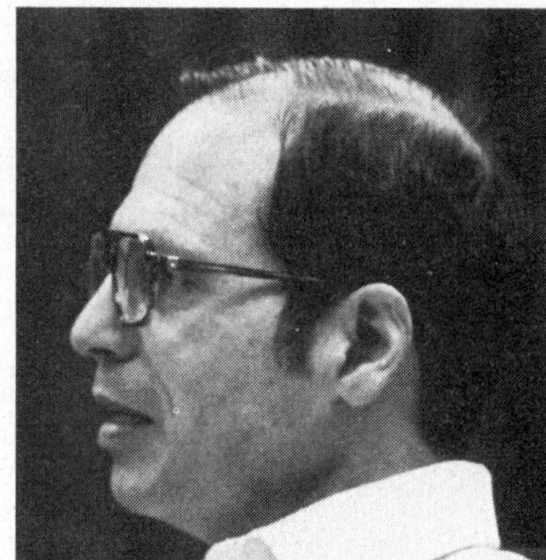

Paul D. Stolley, M.D., M.Ph.

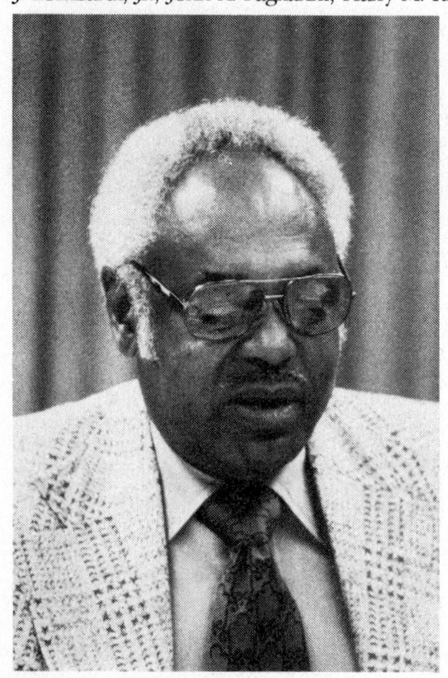

Clifton A. Cole, M.P.A.

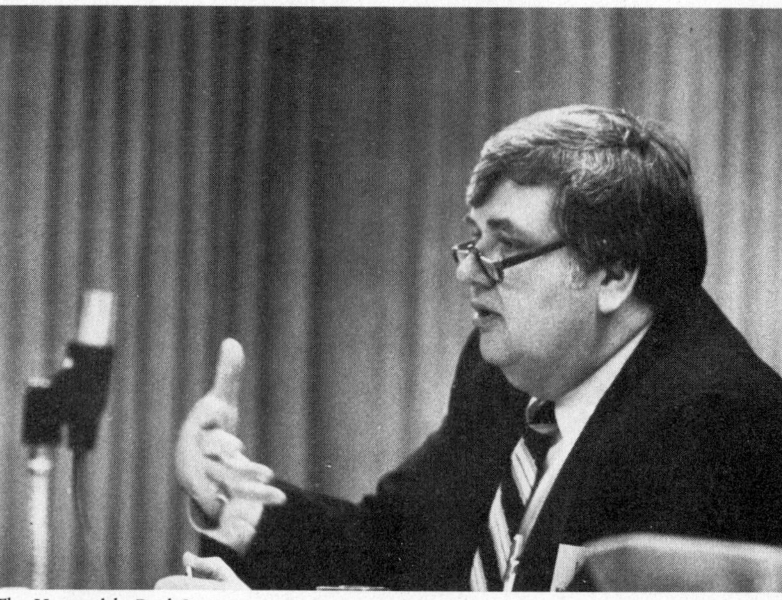

The Honorable Paul Starnes

Photos: Janis R. Nollendorfs

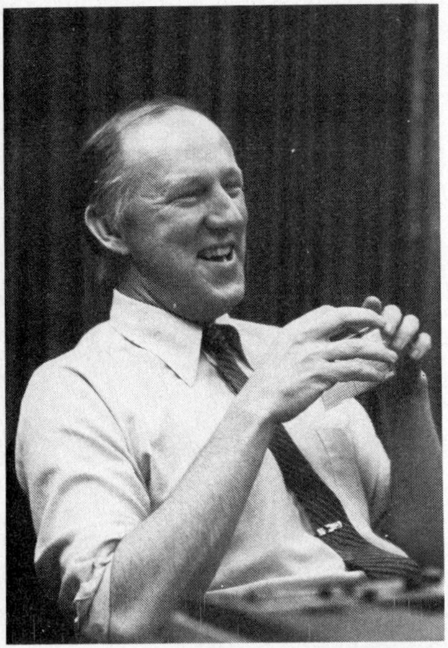

Duncan Neuhauser, Ph.D.

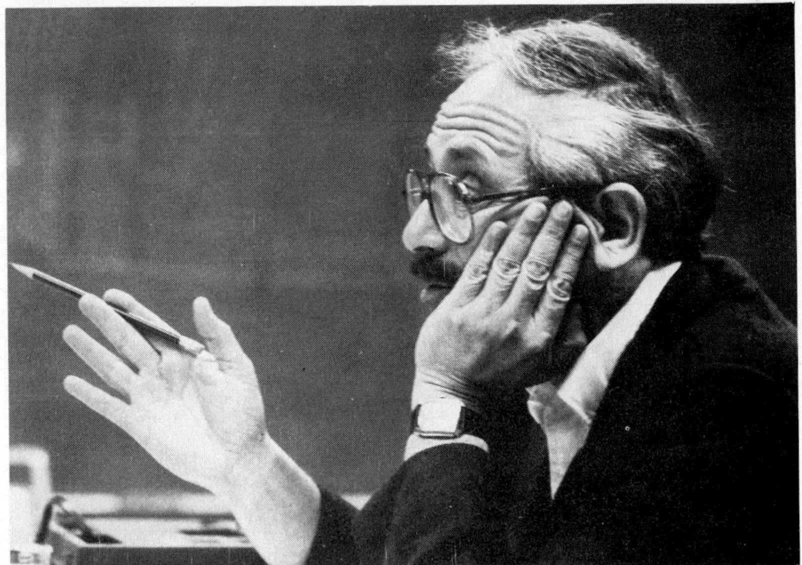

Sumner Robinson, Ph.D.

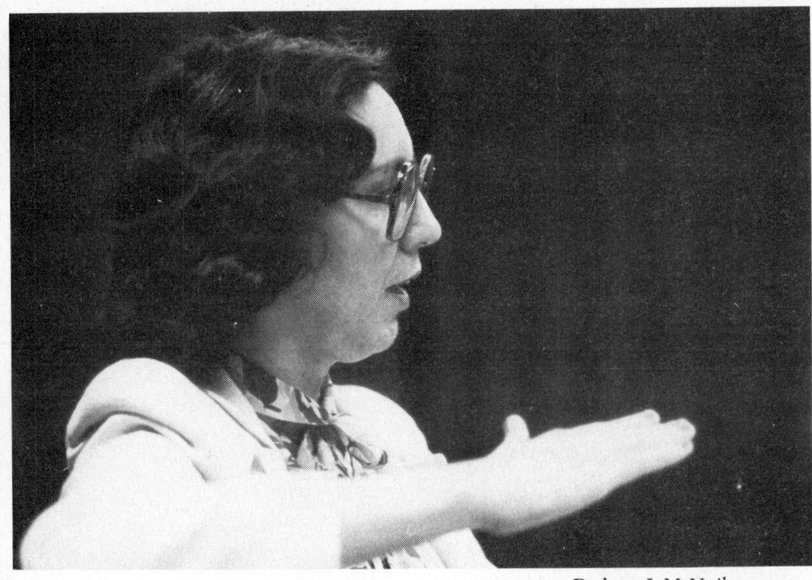

Barbara J. McNeil, M.D., Ph.D.

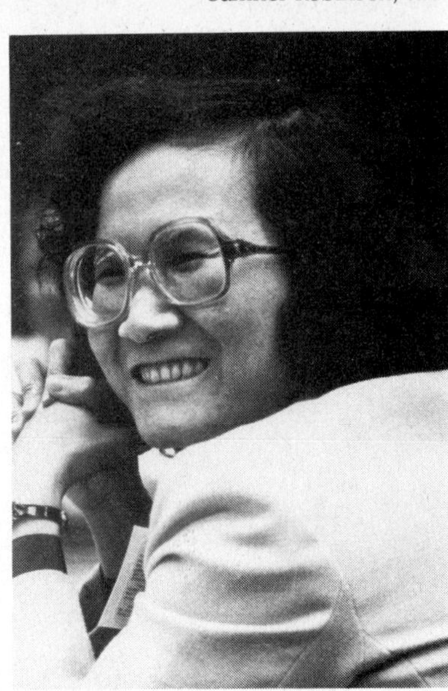

Thi D. Dao, Ph.D.

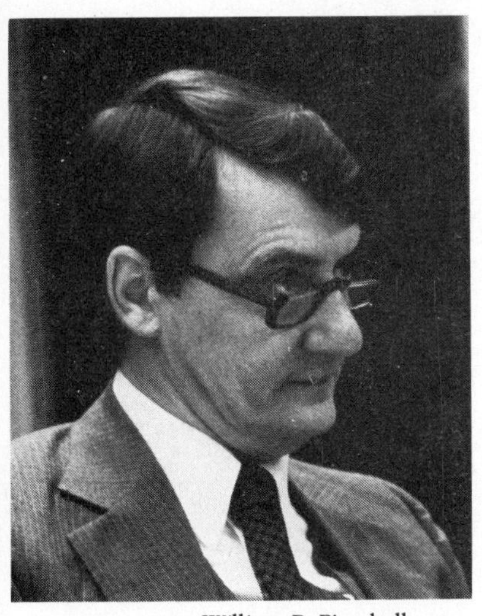

William P. Pierskalla, Ph.D.

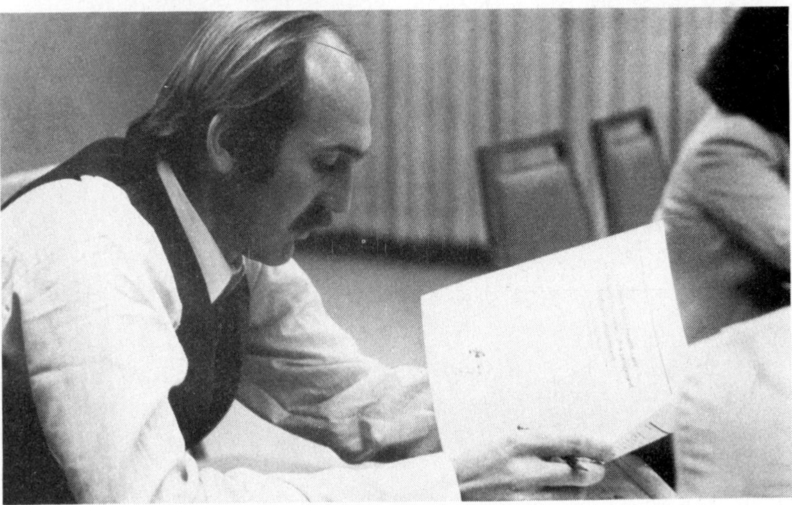

Vernon K. Smith, Ph.D.

THEME I:
Use of CBA/CEA in Policymaking

Summarized by Harvey V. Fineberg, M.D., Ph.D.

1. From Whose Perspective Are Cost–Benefit and Cost–Effectiveness Analyses Done and Whose Perspective Should Be Used? Who Are the Potential Users?

Cost-benefit and cost-effectiveness analyses (CBA/CEA) have traditionally been applied to public goods, such as defense and water resources. Decisions in the health care field involve both public and private goods, and they affect public as well as private interests.

The three small groups responsible for this theme generally believed that CBA/CEA should be done from a societal perspective. That is, an effort should be made to include all costs and benefits no matter who is affected. A range of disciplinary perspectives, including economics, statistics, epidemiology, and medicine, need to be involved in any health-related CBA/CEA.

The groups discussed the difference between a philosophical-analytical perspective for CBA/CEA and the practical questions concerning the decision-making process. Every prescriptive analysis entails some valued objectives that imply a point of view. The philosophical question then becomes: Whose values and interests should be represented in an analysis? Although the groups agreed that the answer was societal interest, practical concerns about the adoption and implementation of the recommendations from CBA/CEA must consider the interests, values, and objectives of decision makers and affected parties. An objective of analysis, therefore, might be to reinforce societal values and their role, which are also a part of what decision makers have to consider.

Speculation arose that we may be entering a period of attempts at rapid adoption of new therapies on the one hand, while on the other, tempered by cost restraints, attempts will be made to make cost-effectiveness data even more influential. Medical care is faced with the question of how to define, gather, and disseminate CBA/CEA data with the introduction of new technology. Obviously, data generated for efficacy and safety considerations are the most important factors and must be studied before CBA/CEA will also be considered important, although not necessarily mandatory, for all technologies. The difficulty in doing CBA/CEA and assessing its value varies with the technologies. For example, it can be more easily done for vaccines than for artificial organs.

2. To What Degree do External (Political) Factors Influence Decision Making? How can CBA/CEA Influence or Mitigate These Factors?

Here, too, we are dealing with group participation and interaction. CBA/CEA is one tool available for decision making, although its usefulness is not entirely accepted or proven as yet. In the future, it may be of greater use and importance than at present, but that will depend on its objectivity, credibility, and record for correct predictions.

Another critical factor in dealing with external elements is whether more restrictive medical-care use policies will be adopted at the state level. If more restrictive policies evolve, as many suspect they will, and if the record for CBA/CEA is positive, these data will have an increasingly important role in the decision-making process.

While CBA/CEA researchers are often optimistic about the usefulness of their study results, that optimism often contrasts with extreme caution on the part of the decision maker. The decision maker may have extensive experience with a variety of evaluation tools that have failed or have at least proven unworkable in their particular context.

Finally, CBA/CEA can be utilized as an ongoing measure of program efficiency and effectiveness, working both as a quality control and decision-making mechanism.

3. What Types of Information Are Available to Policymakers? What Types Are Needed?

A number of data sources are available. Much of our current data originate from the Food and Drug Administration or from studies published in the medical literature. Many are not as well-designed, as well-controlled, or as well-analyzed as possible. Studies at the state level emphasized cost or cost saving rather than the balance between benefits and costs. Because of current fiscal concerns, cost studies were expedient and deemed more important over the short term. But it was readily recognized by the small working groups that CBA/CEA will gain dramatically in importance. Cost alone is insufficient without knowledge of program effects or benefits.

4. What Research Result Format Would Be Most Useful to Policymakers?

It was felt that CBA/CEA can influence politicians, legislators, and other decision makers. But more importantly, it would be a mechanism to communicate with special or vested interest groups. Ideally, an assessment should come from independent sources and be credible, authoritative, definitive, and even overwhelming.

Formally written reports would be useful, but information disseminated in seminars, meetings, and conferences could also be extremely valuable. For example, the emphasis should be on bottom-line information that goes directly to the heart of the subject rather than long, verbose reports that lay out every detail in exacting terms. A summary of data, for example, in a medical letter format, would be important to communicate CBA/CEA information and results.

5. If Cimetidine Is a Good Example of Well-Studied Technology, How Were Policy Decisions Influenced by Research Results?

No CBA/CEA data were presented at the time of initial cimetidine marketing. Perhaps this will always be the case, that phase II studies are simply not constructed in ways to generate these data.

Many states had open formularies, and therefore, fewer financial constraints or considerations at the time of cimetidine's introduction. Cimetidine was accepted primarily because of therapeutic considerations and the enthusiasm of the medical community, rather than because of CBA/CEA.

In states that have a formulary, it was felt that CBA/CEA studies were primarily responsible for the adoption of cimetidine. Therefore, CBA/CEA data, which usually follow the time of initial decision making, may influence important secondary decisions. For example, the possibility exists that drugs may be deleted from the formulary as financial constraints increase, or conversely, CBA/CEA may induce inclusion in the state formulary.

THEME II: Integration of Research Results with External Factors in the Policy and Decision-Making Process

Summarized by James T. Doluisio, Ph.D.

1. Construct a Model of the Decision-Making Process(es) for Medical Technology and Specify Where the Use of Research Results Fits in.

The small groups developed three models. A state Medicaid decision-making model depicted decisions made by the governor and legislators through appropriations processes that affected the Medicaid Program (Figure 1). The second model showed the Food and Drug Administration approval process and its effects on those who produce and utilize drugs (Figure 2). The third model generalized the types of information or models needed by various policy decision-making groups (Figure 3).

It was felt that although national data must be credible to be useful, at the same time, states have their own concerns about accuracy and applicability of local data drawn from national data sets. The groups realized that common sense and informal approaches to decision making used in the past are not as relevant today. The future will hold more complex problems and more difficult decisions as more people become involved in the decision-making process. CBA/CEA can have an increased impact in this environment.

The availability of data must be timely, especially if a costly new intervention is proposed to replace a less costly one. Then CBA/CEA, including data on relative cost and efficacy, will be important.

The indirect effects of an intervention will have to be evaluated beforehand if it is to be introduced into a state Medicaid program. The indirect effects of new technologies on other budgets within Medicaid would be extremely important and persuasive information in the final policy determination.

Involved or affected parties include the executive and legislative branches of government, patients and other consumer groups, physicians and health care providers, third-party payers, private industry, and the academic and research community. A useful analysis, then, would include a parallel assessment of the perspectives, problems, and concerns of these decision makers and affected parties.

The groups briefly discussed the difference between prospective analysis, which addresses current decisions, and retrospective analysis, which reviews past decisions. Reviews of previous decisions may provide a benchmark for future analysis and may lead to the appropriate revision of past decisions.

2. What Are the Principal Methodologic Limitations in CBA/CEA for Study of Medical Technology?

The groups did not agree on the definitional differences among methodologic, practical, and perceptual limitations, but some agreement was reached on the important examples and types of limitations. Everyone was aware, for example, of the absence of adequate epidemiologic and clinical data to support CBA/CEA.

One example of a perceptual problem was a failure to address distributional effects of the costs and benefits in analysis. One limitation may be that the analyses are not always acted upon, but this may be a result of an imperfect decision-making process.

The groups also discussed the difference between the analysis per se and the way in which the analysis is presented to the decision maker. The

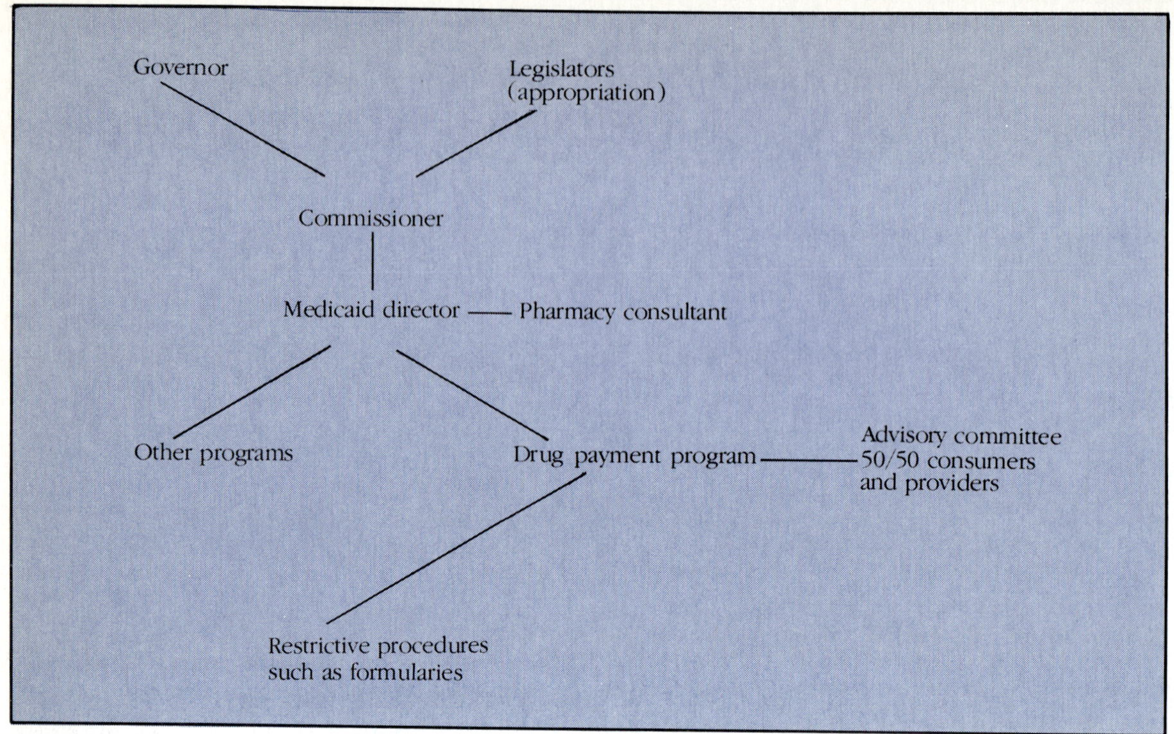

Figure 1. State Medicaid decision-making model.

complexity of the analysis as well as the perspective and requirements of the decision maker require a distinction between the presentation and the substantive issues of the analysis.

The groups discussed other analytic issues. One topic dealt with the idea that any analysis must be presumed to reflect either societal values or the values of those who may be affected by a decision. Another is that adequate and reasonable information about a medical technology must be available before evaluating the effect of CBA/CEA. Third, data are frequently scanty in the early stage in the development of a technology, a time when the decision maker is most eager to have a useful evaluation. On the other hand, an analysis at an early stage can also point out those areas in greatest need of research in making future decisions.

Complementary risks that must be weighed are either a premature decision or one that is made too late. We are always faced with uncertainty in decision making. We can make the mistake of adopting inferior technology that is quickly obsolete or delaying too long the adoption of good technology. The analysis has to thread its way between these two problems.

The world is dynamic with constantly changing circumstances that make analysis difficult. The presently available analysis may not be appropriate for the decision that must be made today and utilized in the future. The analyst may also be restricted by resources and time, preventing a complete analysis of a problem.

There is a tendency to evaluate new rather than extant procedures and to overemphasize this assessment of the new, generally thinking that new is better.

Finally, the existence of vested or special interest groups who have the power to influence decision making can constitute another real problem. The analysis itself may be impolitic or can create other problems ranging from errors of omission to misspecification of either the model or the specifics in the analysis.

3. Are There Other Appropriate Techniques Complementing CBA/CEA for Constrained Decision Making?

Because the focus of the symposium was on CBA/CEA, discussion of alternatives was minimal. In general, other techniques are required to evaluate measures such as provider satisfaction with a program by using informal or intuitive approaches to decision making.

Some discussion was held but no conclusion drawn about using the marketplace as a mechanism for allocating resources rather than current

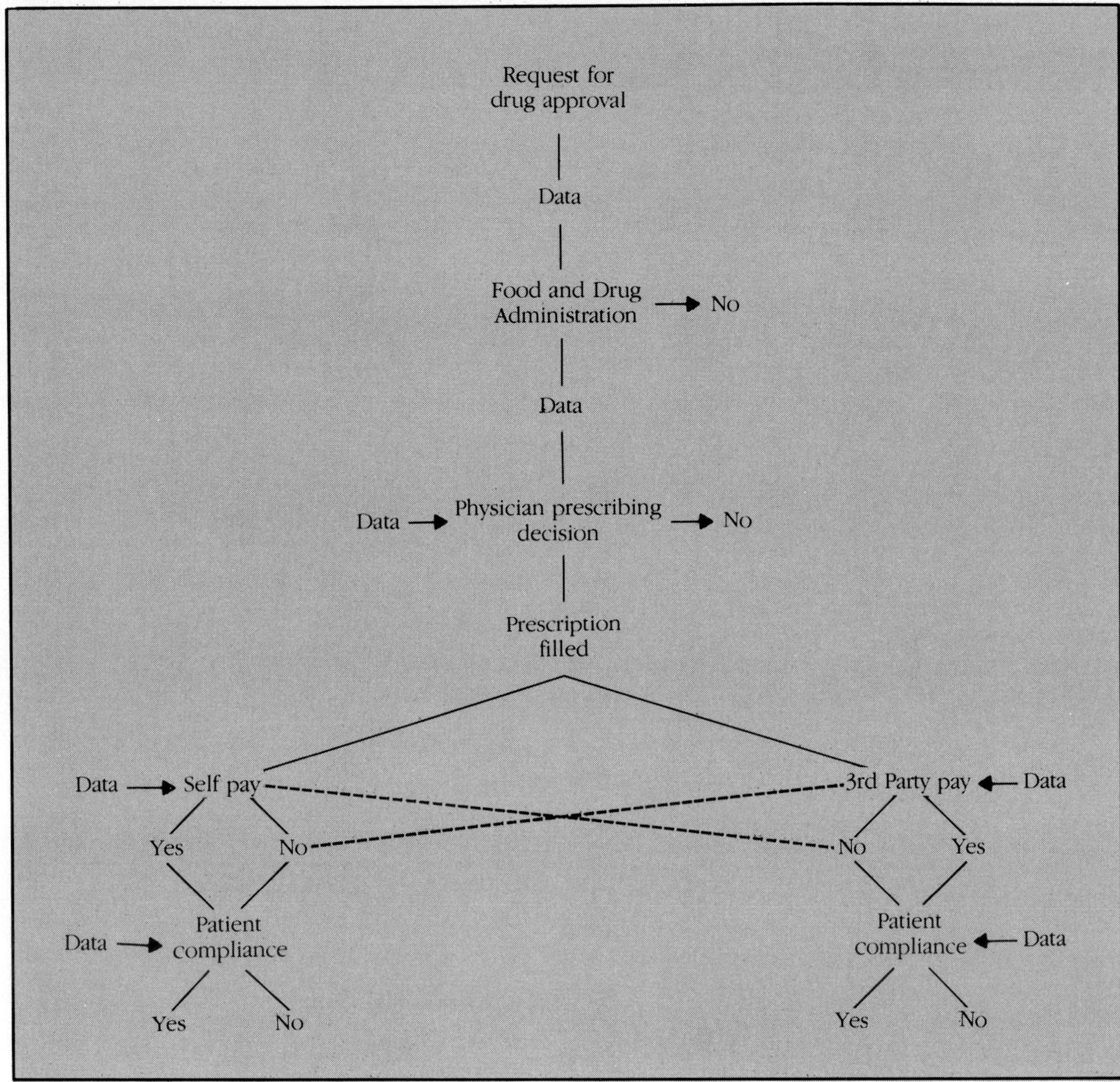

Figure 2. Drug approval — utilization model.

methods and formal evaluative techniques appropriate for this setting.

The example of cimetidine demonstrated the critical importance of combining clinical and epidemiologic studies in the analysis of any new medical technology. CBA/CEA, in fact, could not be done without first submitting to these initial trials. Before cost is considered, effectiveness is the most important criterion.

4. How can CBA/CEA Results be Used in Decision Making?

For any CBA/CEA to be accepted and utilized, the key component must be to assure the credibility of both the analysts and the analysis. The analysis must be based on unbiased information obtained by a well-designed and well-executed study.

Second, prospective users should have more access to analytic results and to producers of needed information.

Third, additional discussion focused on the need to involve the decision maker in the formulation of policy alternatives that are used in the analysis. This is useful even if the decision maker does not necessarily have the same perspective as that of the analyst.

Fourth, advantages may exist in a "quick and dirty" or incomplete analysis when a competent analyst is available to provide incomplete

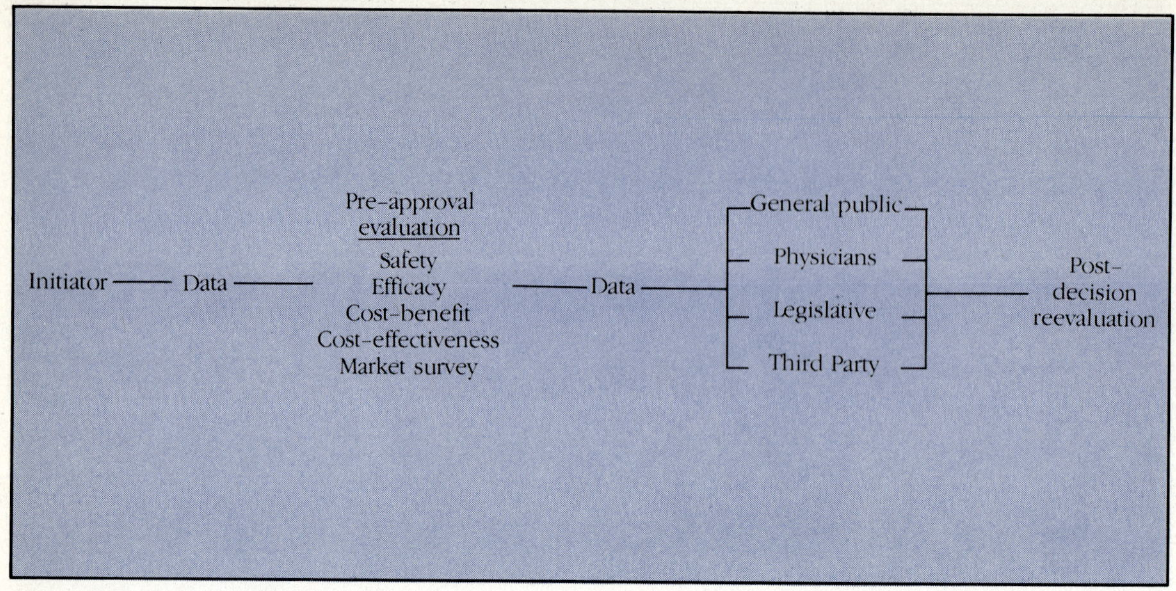

Figure 3. General information model.

information needed quickly. It can point to the direction in which the results of the analysis are heading, and that may be enough to make a decision.

Fifth, some discussion ensued about the training of policymakers to make better choices when commissioning an analysis. The objectives of the policymaker are to select the analyst in a more informed manner, to be able to define the question or problem appropriately, and finally, to digest, understand, and utilize the results.

Finally analysts should be fully informed about the particular needs and perspectives of various decision makers and about political influences so that they are better able to apply their techniques. For example, physicians should have a better grasp of the basic analytic methods so that they can be more informed users of analytic results when making diagnostic and treatment decisions. And patients themselves, acting as informed consumers, should have enough information to interpret the results of the analysis.

5. Cimetidine is an Interesting Case Because Everyone Wins. What About Situations in Which There are Losers as Well as Winners? How Typical is the Cimetidine Model?

There are obviously sharp limits to the general applicability of results for a particular intervention like cimetidine. But, the methodologic application of CBA/CEA to the case of cimetidine was of more general interest.

In particular, some desirable lessons learned from the cimetidine model are:

- The importance of the combination of clinical trials and epidemiological studies in analyzing any new medical technology.
- The importance of identifying the relevant alternatives that must be considered when weighing the costs, benefits, and effects of a particular technology.
- The importance of understanding changes in the evolution of the underlying or natural history of the disease process.
- The problem of what might be called "technology creep," (a given technology, adopted and initially applied for a particuylar use, is applied to increasingly marginally beneficial uses).
- The importance of perspective in the analysis.

The question of who wins and who loses comes up sharply in the case of cimetidine, whether viewed from the perspective of a particular third-party payer for pharmaceuticals, a third-party payer interested in all health costs, or a societal decision maker interested in total health implications. The question, then, of who wins and who loses also carries us back to our point of departure: From whose perspective should the analysis be carried out?

THEME III:
Priorities for Future Studies of Medical Technology

Summarized by Clifton A. Cole, M.P.A.

1. How can CBA/CEA be Made More Useful for Policy and Planning Decision Makers?

These three working groups concluded that CBA/CEA are not the only studies needed. They are only one set of available techniques that need to be coupled with other methodologies for more complete answers to decision-making problems.

It was concluded that retrospective data, which CBA/CEA usually utilize, are not always the best. It is important to use CBA/CEA at the start of medical technology evaluation.

Cimetidine provides an excellent example of medical technology evaluation, since a multitude of clinical, epidemiological, and CBA/CEA data have been gathered. The model constructed for cimetidine should be applied to other similar problems that can be studied using the same method.

One major deficiency was noted: To date, evaluation of the effects of patient education on consumer behavior have not been thoroughly examined. Patient health education, therefore, might be included in future CBA/CEA analyses and evaluated in a similar manner to other health and medical care services.

2. What Information Gaps Would Effectively Realize the Full Potential of CBA/CEA? How Should These Gaps be Filled? What Types of Studies (Methodological/Substantive) Need to be Conducted?

Since existing data do not provide policy analysts with enough information to evaluate medical technology, studies should be planned and implemented during the initial planning stages of a technology. At the other end of the research spectrum, follow-up studies could determine if the original outcomes were obtained. For example, a follow-up study of cimetidine might demonstrate efficacy in other diseases. Additional study may even be necessary to further define the drug's role or application. More time as well as further study and analysis are usually needed to clarify these issues once medical technology has been introduced.

Several factors further affect outcome: *Talent* can be better utilized, the *Treasurer* can be better informed, and the *Time* needed for study can be shortened. In other words, these three "T's" are critical elements in any analysis.

Although specific studies are necessary to measure tangible outcomes, to assess functional outcomes, and to identify broader ranges of outcomes, this group also concluded that a need exists for other studies. Topics requiring additional investigation include ways to select individual drugs, hospitalization priorities, rehabilitation, and in-home supportive services. All can be subjected to CBA/CEA. Substitution assessments are needed to identify still other differences in outcomes. Too often one outcome is given preference, or at least priority, over others because of the political, social, and economic factors involved in public decision making.

CBA/CEA studies of alternative courses of action should be undertaken to determine if budgetary changes are warranted. For example, external factors may change costs from those in the original analysis. Finally, competitive or market mechanisms should be examined to determine whether they have cost-reducing effects.

3. What Will be the Roles of Government and the Commercial Sector in the Future of CBA/CEA? Who Will/Should be Doing These Analyses?

The discussion compared the requirements of government research and analysis with those of the commercial sector. Although marketing demands lead to the initial development of most drugs, medical devices and equipment, how much responsibility for research can government undertake? The government has an interest in research spin-offs that affect medical care, but generally has no commercial interest. Government appears willing, however, both informally and indirectly, to enhance product marketability or the development of commercially viable products. Even with current sharp budgetary reductions, the Federal government will probably continue to fund a broad spectrum of medical care research, including CBA/CEA.

The groups also recognized that both government and private sector perspectives should be incorporated into the early planning, developing, and testing stages of medical technology. This would enhance the ability to determine the technology's full range of effects on consumer health.

4. Would Postmarketing Surveillance Aid Decision Makers in Creating Better Long-Range Policies?

Postmarketing surveillance of medical technology may reveal either positive or negative unsuspected effects, reactions, and interactions that could not possibly have been foreseen. Decision makers need this information to re-evaluate their original decisions.

5. To Allocate Resources More Effectively, Can or Should We Find Common Effectiveness Measures for Various Technologies When an Effective Market Is Lacking?

The groups agreed that various government agencies and the private sector should collaborate in the planning and execution of medical technology evaluations. By doing this, criteria for evaluation, outcome measures, and methodologic concerns can be addressed in order to enhance the development, distribution, and marketing of that technology. Other interested parties, such as private foundations and third-party payers, could also participate by addressing their unique areas of concern.

6. How Can the Intangible Benefits and Liabilities Be Defined and Measured for CBA/CEA?

For CBA and CEA to be evaluated on their effects in aiding policy determination, solid data must be developed and used. Unfortunately, available data are not as strong as they should be.

Lastly, the group questioned whether the outcomes obtained by the CBA/CEA studies were worth the efforts expended. Is it worth the time, talent, and money to perform CBA/CEA studies? Have they made a difference in policymaking? Will they make a difference in the forseeable future? To enhance the usefulness of tomorrow's technology, the group felt that these studies should consider society, the individual, governments, and third–party payers—all of the groups with a vested interest.

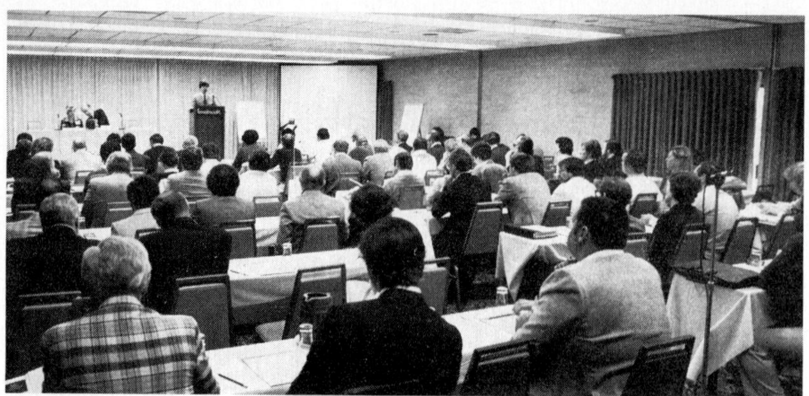

Bernard S. Bloom, Ph.D. addressing conference

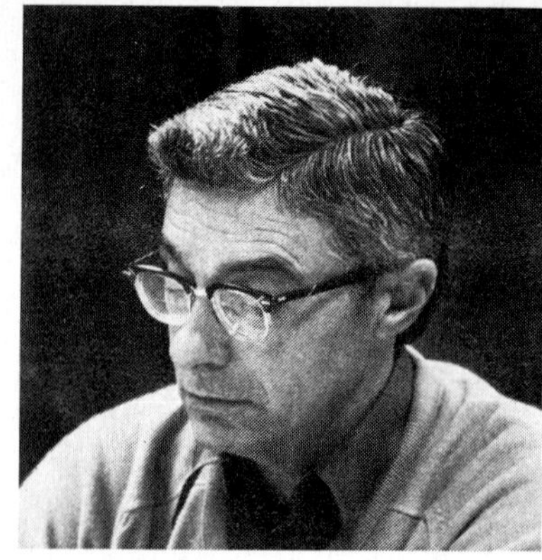

James T. Doluisio, Ph.D.

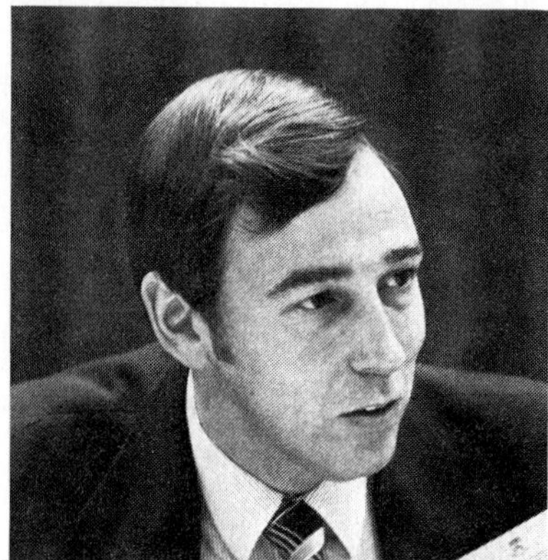

Robert W. Piepho, Ph.D.

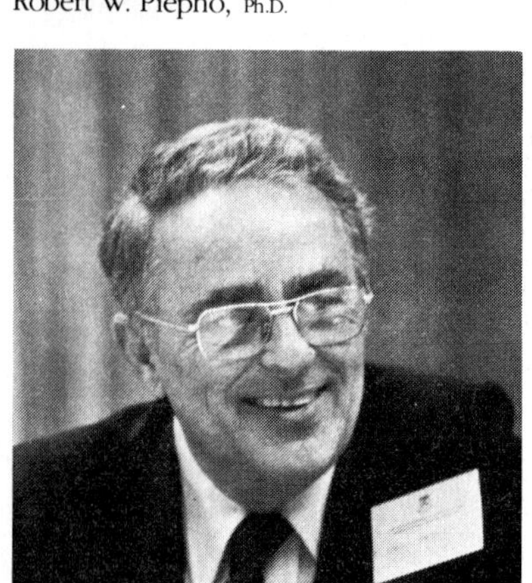

The Honorable Tarkey J. Lombardi, Jr.

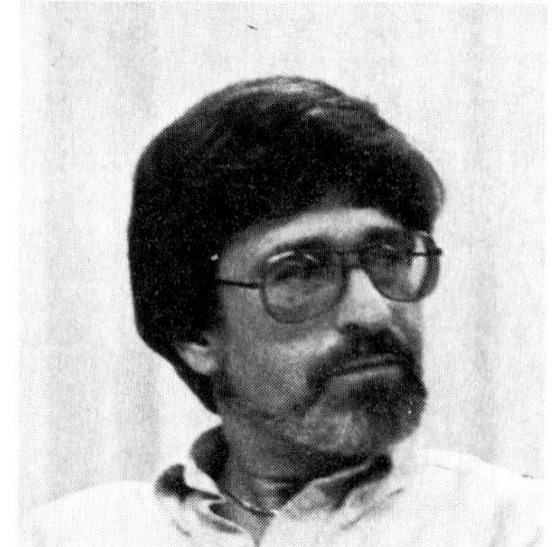

Sanford Luger, R.Ph.

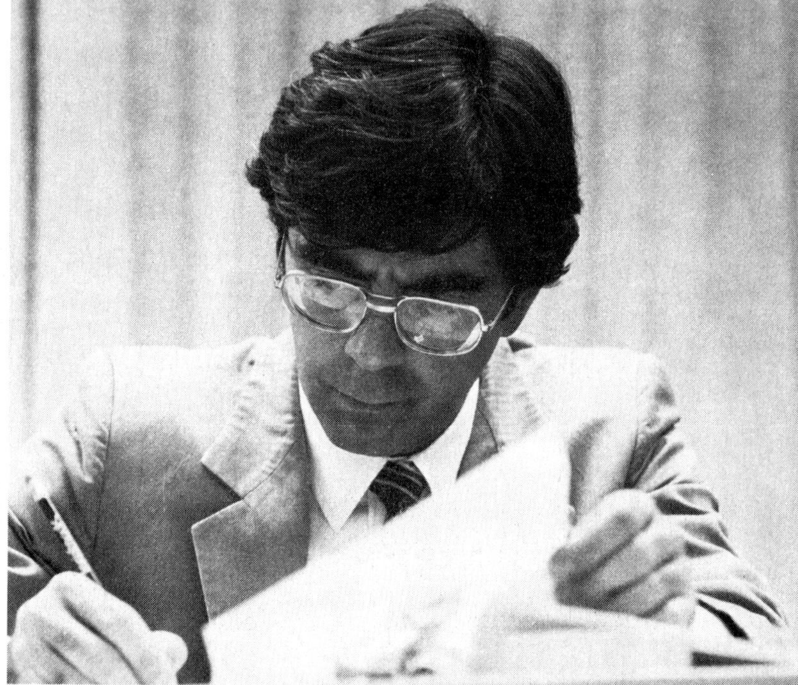

Bernard S. Bloom, Ph.D.

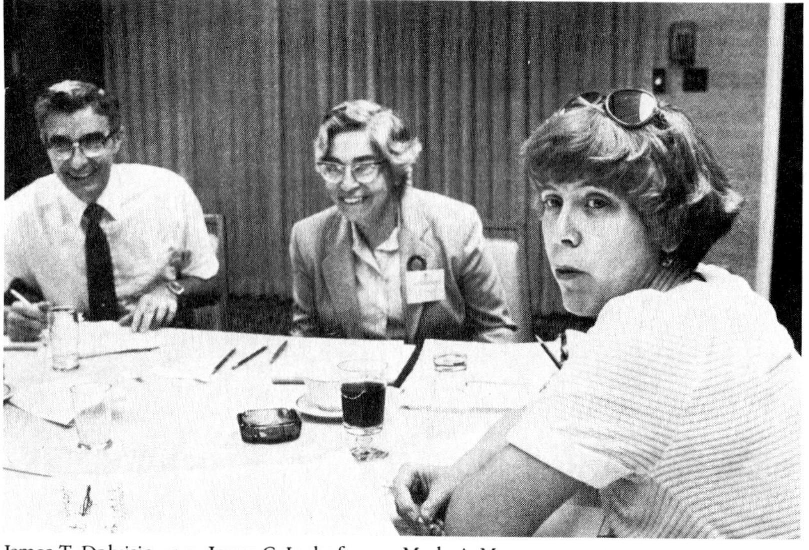

James T. Doluisio, Ph.D.; Joyce C. Lashof, M.D.; Myrle A. Myers, R.Ph.

Photos: Janis R. Nollendorfs

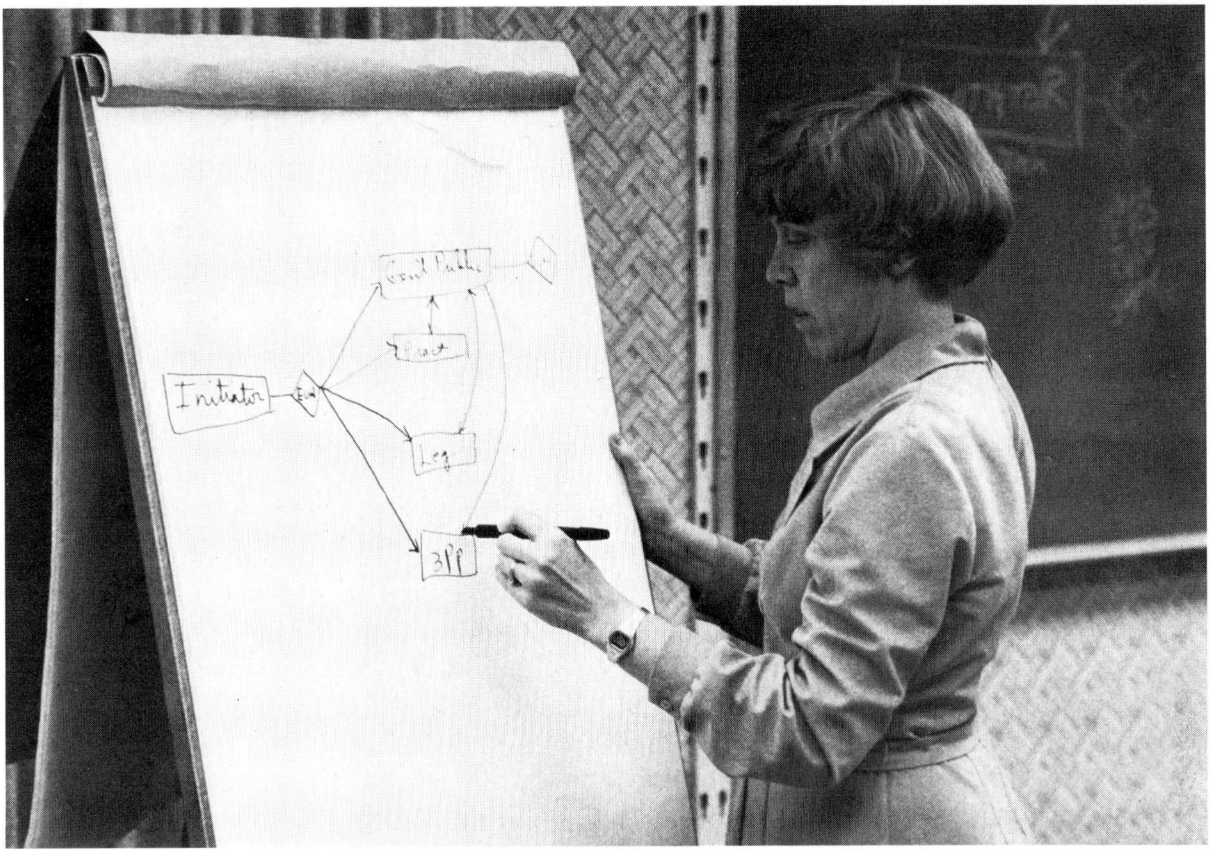

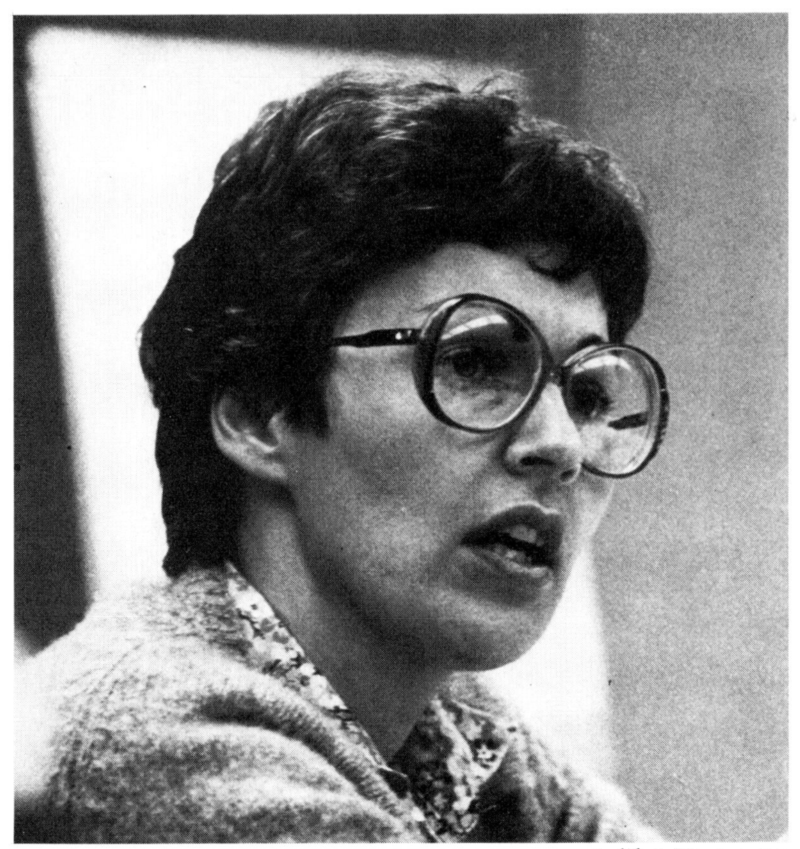

Myrle A. Myers, R.Ph. drawing flow chart during a working group session

Judith L. Wagner, Ph.D.

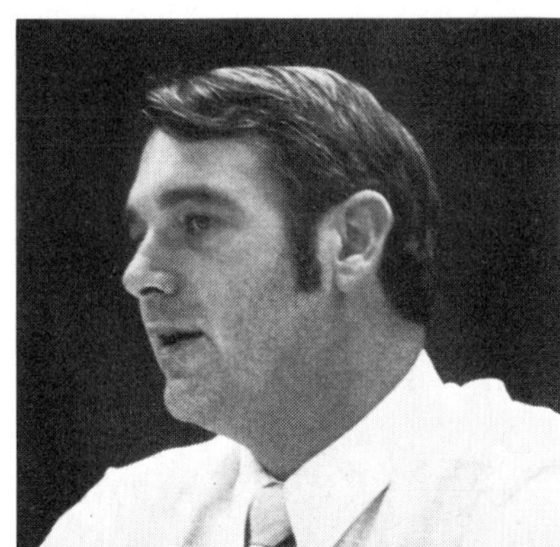

John T. Skhal, Pharm.D.

Arthur E. Cocco, M.D.

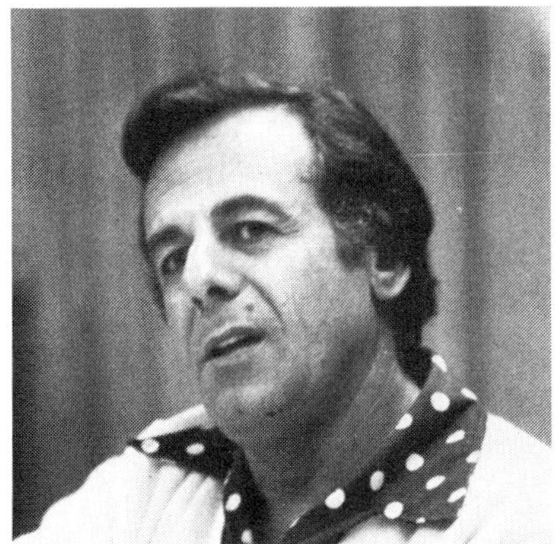

CHAPTER IV
Closing Remarks

Closing Remarks

William P. Pierskalla, Ph.D.

The input and ideas from this conference have been both interesting and productive. I would like to thank the program administrators, analysts, providers, legislators, corporate representatives, and other decision makers for their heterogeneous and unique perspectives. I would also like to thank our speakers for presenting such stimulating talks, and the facilitators for leading our long discussions and synthesizing the results.

If anyone in addition to myself has gained useful insights from this conference, and is now able to make even more meaningful decisions or do better analyses, we have succeeded in what we have tried to do.

Duncan Neuhauser reminded me that we really have to look at the winners and losers in our analyses. The stakeholder analysis is important in anything we do as we often leave out some important stakeholders.

Joyce Lashof impressed me with the complexity of the Federal agency involvement in technology assessment and the extensive assessment that we have put into the investigation process to make better decisions.

Myrle Myers emphasized the enormous informational needs at the state level. I had thought that at this level, the knowledge and information needed to make tough allocation decisions was available and was somewhat surprised to find that the nature of the political process and the self-interest groups affect this decision process in complicated ways.

Finally, Paul Stolley piqued my research interests with his new and exciting approach to how we might scientifically analyze postmarketing surveillance results. He also raised some other concerns and questions about who benefits from some of these studies, where again we saw the importance of stakeholders analysis.

Background Session on Ulcer Disease: Epidemiology, Diagnosis, and Treatment

Background Session on Ulcer Disease: Epidemiology, Diagnosis, and Treatment

Harvey V. Fineberg, M.D., Ph.D.*

Professor of Health Policy and Management
Center for Analysis of Health Practices
Harvard School of Public Health
Boston, Massachusetts

GENERAL CONSIDERATIONS

Epidemiology

Epidemiology is a discipline concerned with the frequency and distribution of disease in a population. As the epidemiology of a disease changes, the social and economic importance of the disease also changes. Understanding the epidemiology of a condition, such as ulcer disease, becomes important when analyzing the cost-effectiveness and cost-benefit of interventions in the disease.

The exact number of patients with ulcer disease is difficult to determine with any degree of accuracy since many people suffer from dyspepsia at some time or other and relatively few actually have an ulcer. Nevertheless, ulcer disease is a common phenomenon. In the United States, 1 of 10 males will suffer from peptic ulcer disease, which includes duodenal and gastric ulcer, at some point in their lives.[1] Approximately 200,000 people in the United States each year develop a new duodenal ulcer, and about 50,000 develop a new gastric ulcer.[2]

The incidence of ulcer disease varies with age and sex. Walker[3] combined data from autopsy studies and clinical surveys and reported an increasing incidence of duodenal ulcer with advancing age, especially among males. Men are generally more prone to this disease than women.

As shown in Figure 1, the incidence of duodenal ulcer in men tends to increase until the mid- to late-40s, peaks around age 50, levels off, and then increases slightly after age 60.[4] Death from ulcer disease is rare, but it is a disease of relatively high morbidity.

Decline in ulcer deaths and hospitalization. The dramatic decline in deaths from ulcer disease in the United States from the mid-1960s up until the late 1970s is an important factor to consider when analyzing the costs and benefits of treatment for ulcer disease. After adjusting for age, the death rate has fallen by more than two thirds from its peak in the mid-1950s until the late 1970s to a level that is now below 2 per 100,000 deaths. As measured by the discharge diagnoses of patients with ulcer disease in the United States, the decline in rates of hospitalization with ulcer disease as the primary cause has accompanied this decrease in the death rate.[5]

Pathology

A duodenal ulcer begins as a shallow erosion in the mucosal tissue, usually in the bulbar area of the duodenum. The ulcer itself is a crater, which extends down the muscle layer of the duodenum. Usually, these ulcers are about 1 to 1.5 cm in diameter—about 50% are smaller than 2 cm in diameter. Occasionally, the ulcer may penetrate through all layers of the duodenal wall, resulting in a perforation. The location and size of a duodenal ulcer are shown in Figure 2.

Although the incidence of duodenal ulcer is more frequent than that of gastric ulcer, they often

---

* Portions of this presentation are adapted from Bardhan KD: Duodenal Ulcer: A current medical perspective. Philadelphia, SmithKline Corporation, 1978.

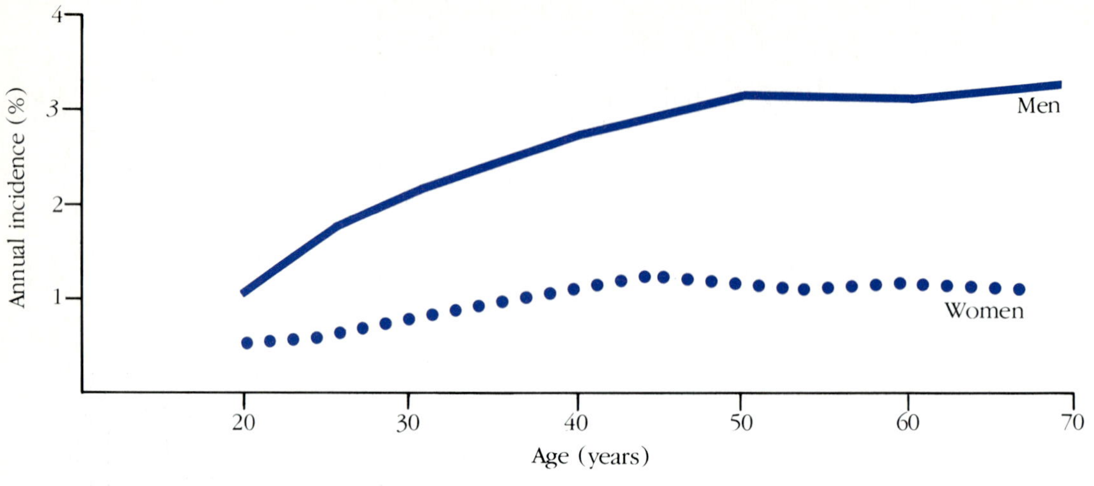

Figure 1. Patterns of Incidence of Duodenal Ulcer Disease According to Age and Sex[2]

coexist. Depending on patient selection and diagnostic method, the occurrence of combined ulcers has been estimated to be between 6 and 65%.[6,7] The cause of such frequent association is unknown.

Complications

Complications of ulcer disease, which may accompany the first or recurrent incidences are usually of three types: hemorrhage, perforation and penetration, and pyloric stenosis.

Hemorrhage. Hemorrhaging or bleeding from either a major artery or smaller vessels in granulation tissue is present in about 20 to 25% of patients with ulcer disease. The most common cause of upper gastrointestinal bleeding is ulcer disease. which accounts for approximately one third of all cases.[8] Bleeding may be only a minor complication, but when the affected blood vessel becomes embedded in fibrous tissue and thus prevents contraction of the eroded edges, the bleeding can become severe. In patients with recurrent and profuse bleeding, mortality may be as high as 15 to 20%.[4,9]

Penetration and perforation. A perforated ulcer is one that has eaten its way through all the layers of the duodenal wall and has actually insinuated itself into the body cavity or backward into the organs. Penetration or perforation are signs of a virulent, aggressive duodenal ulcer but adhesions and penetration are more common. The organ affected is usually the pancreas, which is often directly behind the ulcer. About 5 to 10% of patients will develop a free perforated ulcer; of

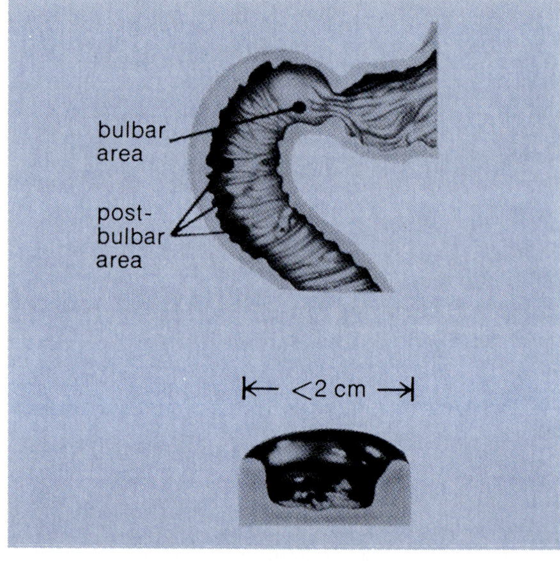

Figure 2. Location and size of duodenal ulcers.

these, over 90% occur on the anterior wall of the duodenum, as this area is not contiguous with other structures. Ulcers on the posterior wall rarely produce such free perforation.

Pyloric stenosis. Repeated insults of inflammation and scarring from attacks of an aggressive ulcer may cause the pyloric channel, the outlet from the stomach into the duodenum, to become stenotic or narrowed. This complication occurs predominantly (over 80%) in men.

Etiology

Imbalance of opposing physiological forces. The exact cause of duodenal ulcer is not known. As a simple explanation, the cause can be considered to be the result of an imbalance between those forces that attack the gastric or duodenal mucosa and those forces that defend the mucosa against attack. Attacking forces comprise gastric acid, pepsin, and possibly bile, whereas the defending forces comprise the mucus covering the gastroduodenal mucosa and the inherent resistance of the duodenal mucosa to attack by acid. In the healthy individual, these forces are considered to be in balance. In the person with ulcer disease, the balance is upset by either an increase in the attacking forces or a decrease in the defending forces (Figure 3).

The balance can be changed by such factors as heredity, environment (ie, diet such as coffee and alcohol intake, and personal habits, such as cigarette smoking), chemicals, drugs, and personality. Why an imbalance initially occurs, why it expresses itself at a particular location, and why some individuals repeatedly experience active attacks are not known.

The role of acid. The importance of acid in normal bodily functions and its role in ulcer formation deserve emphasis. Hydrochloric acid, which is necessary for digestion, is produced by the parietal cells of the stomach, which comprise the largest portion of the stomach's surface. This acid is secreted in response to three kinds of stimuli: nerve excitation, food, and chemicals. For example, sniffing the aroma of food can stimulate the vagus nerve which in turn stimulates the parietal cells to produce acid. The nerve can also cause other cells of the stomach to produce gastrin, a chemical that further stimulates acid production. Once food is eaten, the stretching of the stomach also produces additional acid secretion. When food enters the duodenum, another mechanism is triggered to release even more acid to complete the digestive process. Histamine plays an important part in this process since it facilitates the effects of other chemical stimulators of acid release and probably has a direct role in stimulating gastric acid production. The role of histamine becomes important when considering treatment with cimetidine which will be explained later.

CLINICAL VIEW
Diagnosis

The diagnosis of duodenal ulcer disease is dependent upon the patient's history, physical examination, and diagnostic testing. The diagnosis of ulcer disease is made when the patient presents with either hemorrhage or perforation for the first time. Bleeding may be the first and only presentation that leads to this diagnosis.

Clinical Picture

The predominant symptoms associated with ulcer disease are abdominal pain, vomiting, food intolerance, and occasionally constipation. The symptoms may last for a few days or weeks and then disappear for weeks or months at a time only to reappear again. The clinical picture of duodenal ulcer disease is summarized in the Table.

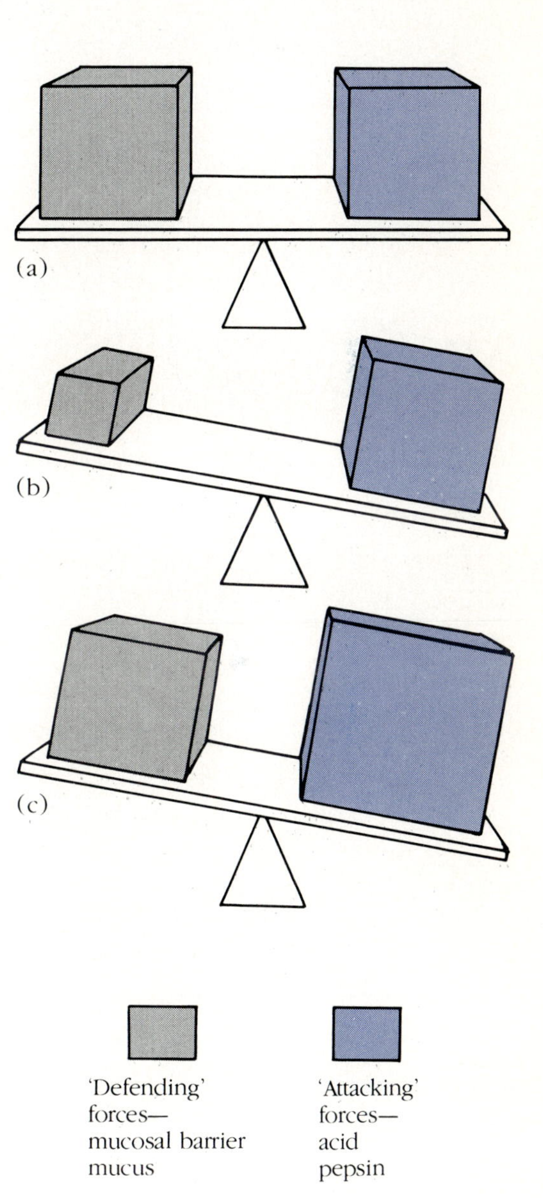

Figure 3. In the healthy individual the 'attacking' and 'defending' forces are presumed to be in balance (a). If this balance is upset either by a decrease in the resistance of the duodenal mucosa (b) or an increase in acid output (c), an ulcer may result.

Table

The Clinical Picture in Duodenal Ulcer Disease

Symptom/Sign	Most usual pattern	Other patterns
Pain		
Location	Upper abdomen, generally in the epigastrium in the midline or sometimes to the right	Above or across the umbilicus Right or left hypochondrium Iliac fossae or groin
Radiation	Upwards toward the retroxiphisternal area or through to the back (midline, between the scapulae)	Away from the epigastrium to both hypochondria, deep to the costal margins From hypochondria through to the back Downwards, in broad, ill-defined band or sharply demarcated narrow zone toward the sub-umbilical area
Nature	General discomfort; descriptions vary from deep, dull, and boring to sharp and cutting	Gnawing, clamp-like, twisting, tearing
Nocturnal pain	"Accentuated hunger pain" Usually occurs between 1:00 and 3:00 AM, irrespective of time of the evening meal or of going to bed	On awakening in the morning
Effect of food	Temporary relief of pain in 50–70% of patients	Increase in pain (see also food intolerance)
Vomiting	Occurs in about 25% of patients with uncomplicated bulbar duodenal ulcer Symptoms of reflux in 75% of patients	Occurs frequently in patients with ulcer close to pylorus with outlet obstruction Occurs frequently when pain is severe Mild vomiting with nausea early in the morning
Food intolerance	Common in active ulceration; fried foods, pastries, cucumbers, curry, onions, are frequent offenders	Wide variety of other foodstuffs to which individual patients may be susceptible
Effect of stress	Recurrence of exacerbation of symptoms, principally "discomfort" and reflux	
Weight loss	Mild and transient when ulcer is active; most common in patients with food intolerance and vomiting	As much as 12 kg during an acute attack
Abnormalities on examination	Mild to moderate epigastric tenderness	Severe epigastric tenderness with guarding
Periodicity of symptoms	Relapsing and remitting pattern; symptoms prominent for 2–4 weeks; remissions lasting 1–3 months.	Symptoms prominent for only a few days or for as long as 8–10 weeks Seasonal variations
Patterns of remission and relapse	Mild, short-lived symptoms occurring initially at infrequent intervals; with time, relapses become more frequent, and more severe, and may last longer or Symptoms remain mild and infrequent for several years, followed by severe attack and rapid deterioration	Frequency of attacks does not change Initial severe attack followed by asymptomatic period that may last for years, followed by recurrence of usually mild symptoms

From Bardhan KD: Duodenal Ulcer: A current medical perspective. Philadelphia, SmithKline Corporation, 1978.

Pain. The hallmark of ulcer disease is pain located in the middle region of the upper stomach, the so-called epigastric region, or sometimes in the right quadrant. The pain may also radiate upward or through to the back where it is felt in the midline between the scapulae. When asked to locate the pain, the patient will often put a hand across the general area of the upper abdomen, but will point in a single area to show where the pain is greatest. The pain most typically occurs in the middle of the night, but occasionally may appear in the morning and is generally relieved by antacids and sometimes by food.

The description of the pain varies widely ranging from deep, dull, and boring to a more sharp and cutting type; other descriptions include a gnawing sensation, accentuated hunger pain, a general burning sensation, or an "air-lock," which is sometimes relieved by belching.

Vomiting. Frequency of vomiting depends on the location of the ulcer; it often occurs when pain is severe, and frequently relieves symptoms. Some patients will induce vomiting because it offers more complete and sustained relief than the usual forms of medical treatment.

Food intolerance. Intolerance to certain foods is a common feature of ulcer disease. Fried foods and pastries are cited by most patients, although a wide range of foods can be potential offenders. Since the intolerance may continue after the ulcer has healed, many patients continue to restrict their diet.

Patterns of remission and relapse. The course of ulcer disease is marked by remissions and recurrences. The length of an individual attack varies. In up to 50% of the cases, symptoms are prominent for 2 to 4 weeks; in others, the attack lasts for only a few days or sometimes, 8 to 10 weeks. Most patients experience at least one relapse within 5 years of an initial ulcer episode. In some chronic cases, the remission period may be less than a month.

The pattern of remission and relapse varies but can be broadly classified into four types:

1. Mild, short-lived symptoms occurring initially at infrequent intervals is more common; with time, relapses become more frequent and last longer.

2. Mild and infrequent symptoms for years, then sudden severe attack with rapid deterioration which may coincide with penetration.

3. Frequency of attacks unchanged; no steady deterioration.

4. Severe initial attack requiring hospitalization after which patient remains asymptomatic until recurrence of less severe symptoms; thereafter, any of first three patterns may develop.

Imaging Procedures

Specific diagnosis of ulcer depends on imaging examinations, such as endoscopy or barium meal, which can detect and demonstrate the presence of an ulcer.

Radiology. Diagnosis of a duodenal ulcer by x-ray can be made only by demonstrating an ulcer crater, or, if none is visible, by finding moderate to marked deformity of the duodenal cap. Adequate technique requires distention of the duodenal cap and coating of the mucosal surface with barium so that all details of the bulb contour and mucosal pattern can be studied. This can be done by using a double-contrast technique that involves both barium and air.

Endoscopy. Endoscopy allows the gastroenterologist to directly visualize the ulcer. Changes are visible not only in the duodenum, but also in the pylorus, antrum, and esophagus.

A normal duodenum seen by endoscopy is shown in Figure 4; Figure 5 shows a duodenal ulcer. The ulcer appears yellowish, irregular, about one-half to one inch in diameter, with quite a bit of inflammation around it. The edges are often irregular. Erosions usually exist with the ulcer and have the same appearance as the ulcer except that they are smaller and more superficial. They may

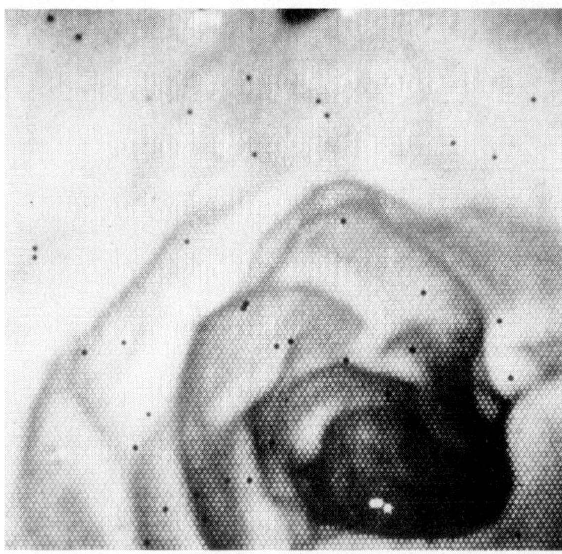

Figure 4. A normal duodenum.

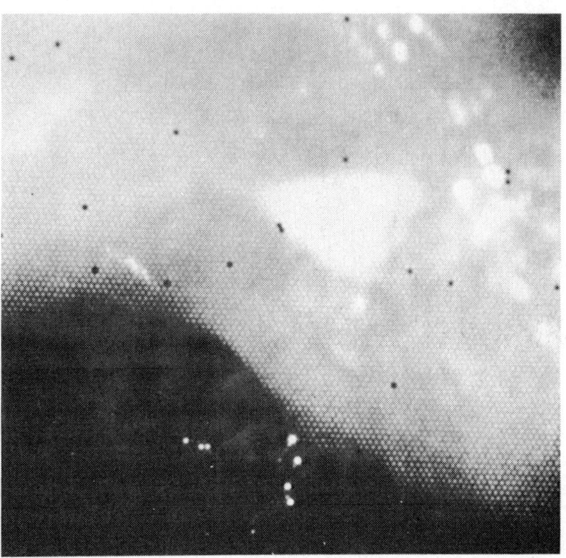

Figure 5. A duodenal ulcer.

surround the ulcer, be scattered, or may occur in groups on the inflamed mucosa.

A healing ulcer may appear flatter and become whitish and smaller in size, with diminished inflammation. Eventually the ulcer may disappear leaving a pale yellow scar although the inflammation takes longer to disappear.

TREATMENT

Aims

If left untreated, most ulcers will eventually heal in 10 to 12 weeks even with little specific treatment. Nevertheless, this period may be one of great discomfort for the patient who may be nearly incapacitated and certainly not able to function normally. The object is then to promote healing at a more rapid rate, prevent recurrences and complications, and, above all, to relieve pain.

All treatments are ultimately aimed at interdicting the effects of gastric acid on the mucosa of the duodenum or stomach, for example, by reducing or neutralizing acid secretion or by increasing the tissue's defenses against the acid.

Diet

Patients are primarily advised to avoid those foods that exacerbate the symptoms (most of which they will probably already know), maintain a regular diet, and avoid coffee, tea, cigarettes, and alcohol. A sufficient amount of rest seems to promote general healing.

Surgery

Surgery is primarily limited to cases in which there are complications or difficulties with medical management.

A variety of surgical approaches are designed to prevent and reduce the amount of acid produced by the stomach. This is accomplished either by eliminating the acid-producing cells through partial gastrectomy or by eliminating the nervous stimulation of gastric acid by vagotomy. Since the vagus nerve is also important in promoting drainage of the stomach contents, some type of drainage procedure is also necessary along with vagotomy. Some surgeons choose to perform more selective vagotomies that sever only those segments of the nerve adjacent to the stomach.

Medications

Antacids, anticholinergics, and cimetidine are the medications now primarily used. Antacids reduce

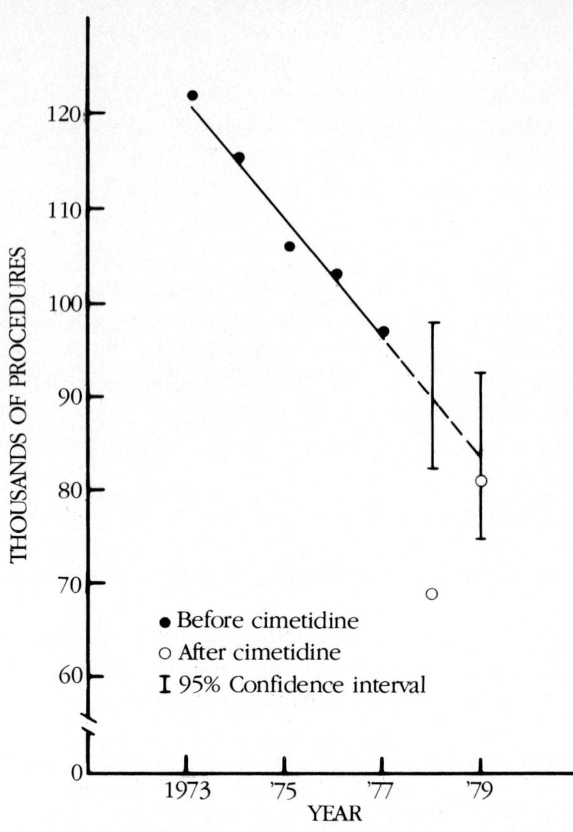

Figure 6. Partial gastrectomy and vagotomy surgery in the United States, 1973-79.

the acidity of the stomach contents. Anticholinergics intervene in the neurostimulation of acid secretion, but have a secondary role in treatment.

Cimetidine

Cimetidine is a drug that was specifically sought to prevent and treat ulcer disease. When it became known that histamine has a central role in the secretion of stomach acid, compounds were developed that actually prevented the histamine stimulation of gastric acid. Because the chemical structure of cimetidine is so similar to histamine, cimetidine fools the body by occupying histamine receptors but without the stimulating effect. Cimetidine prevents approximately 80% of the basal acid output and up to 70% of the stimulated output of gastric acid.

When cimetidine was introduced in the United States in August 1977, it was enthusiastically greeted by physicians in this country. In the year after cimetidine's introduction, the rates of surgery dropped much more than would have been expected by the best linear regression prediction of the surgery rates in the preceding years (Figure 6). This is the kind of evidence that is looked at when analyzing the consequences of medical intervention, and the role that cost-effectiveness analysis plays in the evaluation of new medical practices.

REFERENCES

1. Mendeloff AI: What has been happening to duodenal ulcer? *Gastroenterology* 67:1020, 1974

2. Sturdevant RAL, Walsh JH: Duodenal ulcer. In Sleisenger MG, Fordtron JS (eds): *Gastrointestinal Disease.* Philadelphia, WB Saunders, 1978, 2nd ed.

3. Walker CO: Chronic duodenal ulcer. In Sleisenger MH, Fordtran JS (eds): *Gastrointestinal Disease.* Philadelphia, WB Saunders, 1973, p 669

4. Johnston SJ et al: Epidemiology and course of gastrointestinal haemorrhage in north-east Scotland. *British Medical Journal* 3:655, 1973

5. Fineberg HV, Pearlman LA. Surgical treatment of peptic ulcer in the U.S.: Trends before and after the introduction of cimetidine. *Lancet* 1:1305, 1981

6. Weisberg H, Jerzy Glass GB: Coexisting gastric and duodenal ulcers. *American Journal of Digestive Diseases* 8:992, 1963

7. Rumball JM: Progressive systemic sclerosis (scleroderma) with esophageal and gastric antral involvement *Gastroenterology* 61:622, 1971

8. Schiller KFR et al: Haematemesis and melaena with special reference to factors influencing the outcome. *British Medical Journal* 2:7, 1970

9. Jones PF et al: Further haemorrhage after admission to hospital for gastrointestinal haemorrhage. *British Medical Journal* 3:660, 1973

APPENDIX B

Introduction to Cost-Benefit and Cost-Effectiveness Analysis

Bernard S. Bloom, Ph.D.

Complex CBA and CEA Problems

William P. Pierskalla, Ph.D.

Introduction to Cost-Benefit and Cost-Effectiveness Analysis

Bernard S. Bloom, Ph.D.

Cost-benefit and cost-effectiveness analyses (CBA/CEA) are neither a cure-all nor an end in themselves. They are not a decision-making method, and cannot provide a complete answer for decision-making problems, nor can they substitute for the keen judgment, wisdom, and understanding of the policymaker. Rather, CBA and CEA are only tools being utilized to aid in decision making—nothing more, nothing less. They provide some of the answers regarding costs, effects, or benefits of particular actions under consideration. But, unfortunately, they do not account for the political, social, and economic environments that policymakers must incorporate into any decision-making calculus.

To be effectively applied, these techniques must depend heavily on good data regarding cost, effects, and benefits. Without good data, solid CBA or CEA cannot be developed. Equally important, the answers they provide must be timely, understandable, and applicable to the problems.

CBA seeks to weigh the costs measured, in dollars and cents, of a particular course of action against the benefits derived, also measured in monetary value. The greater the benefit for a given cost, or the lower the cost for a given benefit, the better the program in relation to others with lower cost-benefit ratios.

Of course, a major problem with CBA is placing monetary value on the costs and, most importantly, on the benefits of a program or intervention. For example, what is the value of a human life, of reduced symptoms, or of increased function? Can they be valued? Most would say yes. But how? And, what value is to be placed on them? How objective can the measurements be?

CEA is similar to CBA in that a monetary value is placed on the cost. The two analytic methods diverge because cost-effectiveness seeks only to enumerate the effects of any particular action or program without attaching any monetary value. The costs are monetarized, but the effects are not. The effects can be defined in terms of increased longevity, symptom or disease reduction, changes in functional status, consumer satisfaction, and a host of other individual, system, or program outcomes. The costs of the program are weighed against its expected effects, without putting a monetary value on those effects.

It is important to understand that CBA, CEA, and technology assessment as aids to policymakers are best utilized in evaluating problems of relatively low complexity, where only a few variables have to be measured, such as the costs and effects or benefits of a hypertension screening program or use of a drug such as cimetidine. It is the classic one physician/one patient model.

These methods do not work well with problems that have many variables, multiple options, or large, complex problems. Those may be in the areas of program trade-offs, resource allocation effects, and the like. When money can be spent in many places but only a certain amount of money is available, one must decide which programs potentially have the largest beneficial effects on a population. Thus, once the analysis must go beyond the relatively simple model, with only two or three variables, more complex techniques, such as decision analysis or operations research, are required.

Complex CBA and CEA Problems

William P. Pierskalla, Ph.D.

Numerous problems cannot be considered when using a simple analysis of costs versus benefits. When allocating a limited budget for certain drugs, diagnostic procedures, or therapeutic medical or surgical interventions, cost-benefit or cost-effectiveness analysis in the narrow sense will probably not indicate how to allocate resources most effectively. We need to deal with costs, revenues, benefits, and effects simultaneously with the inputs, outputs, and system transformations that are occurring in health care delivery. In this broader sense, techniques such as decision analysis, operations research, management science, or other system analysis methods enable us to analyze different relationships among different decisions to be made. The problems and systems for which these techniques are applicable usually have to achieve simultaneous multiple objectives and require prioritizing and sequencing to achieve the objectives. In addition, there are usually multiple alternative solutions and the "best" among these alternatives must be selected.

Because of these complexities, it is diffficult for decision makers to consider a large volume of information, as the human mind can usually process only a limited amount of information, alternatives, and decisions at one time. Also a limited amount of time is available to devote to decision making as most officials are involved in numerous activities and essentially must concentrate on one at a time. When the other activities become critical, decision makers then turn their attention to them.

The amount of information initially available is often only a small fraction of the total that is potentially available. But obtaining that additional information may be costly in terms of time, money, and effort.

Finally, information on important aspects of any problem may be difficult or impossible to obtain and often deals with future events. And yet decisions must be made today to cover those events. Since cost-benefit and cost-effectiveness analyses, in the narrow sense of these terms, cannot handle those complexities of decision making, techniques are needed to combine multiple objectives and constraints on the problem. We must be able to perform "sensitivity analyses" of the problem. That is, we must investigate the decisions that can be made today so that under different scenarios and probabilities of occurrence of future events we will obtain a reasonably good set of decisions. If we look at costs, benefits, and effects in this broader sense, then we can start to solve some of these more difficult problems in evaluating complex technology and its utilization.

To identify the different alternatives to use in more complex decision making, certain information must be obtained. Some of the future conditions or possible scenarios that could evolve must be identified along with the criteria to evalute these alternatives and future scenarios. The probabilities of occurrence must also be assessed. Furthermore, the importance or priorities of the different criteria to be used in the evaluation process must be identified. Techniques such as Delphi, Hierarchical Analysis, Nominal Group, and Conjoint Analysis as well as more formal statistical techniques can be used to gather these probabilities and priorities. Finally, the effectiveness and costs of different alternatives, conditions, criteria, and the constraints to achieve them must be determined.

The broader based evaluative technologies would be able to choose from those alternatives, based on the multiple criteria, in order to determine the best set of decisions that could be made. For example, in screening for different types of cancers, when is it optimal to use certain tests? A large number of tests are available, ranging from patient histories to detailed invasive or noninvasive testing utilizing major technologies. But, these different tests and technologies have different costs, risks, and accuracies. To make decisions about which tests and technologies are appropriate for a particular person at a particular time, you must look at the objectives you are trying to achieve. Do you want, for example, to maximize life expectancy? To maximize the reduction in risk of death at younger ages? To minimize income loss? To minimize the cost of medical treatment? To increase life quality in some dimensions? To reduce fatigue among the people with these characteristics? To reduce emotional stress? These are some of the different objectives to be achieved with prevention programs and the use of modern technologies. Yet how do we assess these technologies in this broader context? All have a first step in that the objectives must be prioritized in a meaningful fashion for either the individual or society. Then a broad based cost and effectiveness analysis utilizing systems analytic techniques must be performed to arrive at which preventive tests are to be applied at which times for different groups of the population at risk. These techniques can either minimize certain of the objectives subject to the achievements of other objectives at some level of acceptability to society.

One of the purposes of this symposium is to assess cost-benefit and cost-effectiveness analysis as technologies in their own right. To do so we must consider the narrow range and capabilities of simple CBA and CEA as well as the broad based system analytic techniques.

Cimetidine Research Summaries: Examples of CBA/CEA

The Cimetidine Studies: Examples of Cost-Benefit Information

The studies are briefly summarized in an order chosen to reveal their various types. Those preceded by an asterisk are particularly noteworthy as examples of different study approaches. (No comment on study quality is implied.)

***1. Cost of Ulcer Disease in the United States, SRI,** 1977.

By defining the direct and indirect costs of disease at the national level—using published national statistics and projections from more limited data—the groundwork is laid for future macroeconomic studies of the impact on those costs of a new medical intervention. The costs in 1977 are estimated to total $3.2 billion, about evenly divided between direct and indirect costs. Hospital care is by far the largest direct cost, morbidity the main indirect cost.

2. The Impact of Cimetidine on the National Cost of Duodenal Ulcers, Robinson Associates, Inc., 1978.

This estimation study, based on interviews with cimetidine clinical investigators prior to market introduction, suggests what economic effects the intervention might have if adopted widely for the disease in question. The investigators' estimations of treatment and response patterns with and without cimetidine were costed out and projected to the national level. It is estimated that the national costs of duodenal ulcer in 1977 would have been reduced by 29% if cimetidine had been used in 80% of duodenal ulcer patients.

***3. Preliminary Methodology for Controlled Cost-Benefit Study of Drug Impact: the Effect of Cimetidine on Days of Work Lost in a Short Term Trial in Duodenal Ulcer,** Ricardo-Campbell et al, 1980

Based on randomized double-blind trials, this study illustrates the value of controlled experimental design in defining the effect of a pharmacologic intervention. Through analysis of work-loss data obtained on a subset of patients during the trials, the definition of efficacy is broadened, with socioeconomic implications. In the subset, patient improvement, as measured by time lost from work, was significantly greater among cimetidine-treated patients than among the placebo-treated controls. The difference was evident by the end of the first week and increased during the 6-week period.

4. Maintenance Treatment of Recurrent Peptic Ulcer by Cimetidine, Bodemar and Walan, 1978.

This study extends controlled experimental observation to one year. To work-loss data, it adds data on ad libitum antacid consumption and extent of hospitalization for surgery. The latter, particularly, broadens the definition of efficacy and has obvious economic implications for the health care system. One out of the 32 patients on cimetidine, versus 15 out of the 36 patients on placebo, needed ulcer surgery. The cimetidine-treated group generated 79 days of lost work because of ulcer versus 1,405 days lost among the placebo group.

5. Socioeconomic Aspects of Treatment with Cimetidine in Peptic Ulcer Disease, Bodemar et al, 1980.

The economic implications of reduced work loss and hospitalization (above) are explored in the context of national costs of the disease. It is recognized that the cost savings of reduced surgery during treatment will be substantially increased if surgery can be avoided over the long-term. Use of long-term treatment will depend on long-term safety.

*6. **Surgical Treatment of Peptic Ulcer in the United States: Trends Before and After the Introduction of Cimetidine,** Fineberg and Pearlman, 1981.

Unlike results from strict, randomized clinical trials (involving select patients, required dosages, and placebo controls), the epidemiologic data in this study reflect natural experience in the community. The rapid and widespread adoption of cimetidine treatment in the U.S. is documented. The possible effect of the new intervention is discerned through trend analysis, with surgery for other diseases used as a control. Compared with prior trend and with other abdominal operations, surgery for ulcer disease shows a striking drop in 1978. This is coincident with the rapid adoption of cimetidine, introduced in the fall of 1977.

7. **Effect of Cimetidine on Surgery for Duodenal Ulcer,** Wyllie et al, 1981.

This brief study illustrates simplified trend analysis of regional data in England. The authors suggest that the number of operations performed provides a meaningful indication of effectiveness. The trend in operations for duodenal ulceration shows a sharp break in 1977, following the introduction of cimetidine in the fall of 1976.

8. **Surgery and Hospitalization Trends in the UK Before and After Cimetidine,** Venables, 1981.

This study illustrates trend analyses of both regional and national data in England. An unexpected drop in surgery with no rebound is seen following the introduction of cimetidine. Distinguishing between elective and relatively infrequent emergency surgery, it finds no trend change in the latter—suggesting no change in the incidence of ulcer disease in the community, only in the frequency of elective surgical treatment.

9. **The Effect of Cimetidine on Peptic Ulcer Disease in Rhode Island,** Rhode Island Health Services Research, Inc., 1981.

Using local Blue Cross and Blue Shield charges for surgical and nonsurgical hospital stays, this study translates the trend change in surgical intervention after introduction of cimetidine into reductions in average hospitalization costs. A national projection is made. In 1978, at the national level, the total savings in hospitalization and physician costs due to decreased surgery is projected at $59 million to $97 million. Some outpatient costs and absenteeism trends are also examined.

*10. **Cimetidine-Related Findings by the Netherlands Economic Institute,** Bulthuis, 1981.

Based on 8 years of national data, this work uses multiple regression analysis to isolate the contribution of trend, endoscopy, cimetidine, and other variables to a pronounced decline in the relative cost of treating ulcer disease. Increased drug costs are considered in the light of considerably reduced hospital costs and a net effect calculated. A net saving from cimetidine of 4.5 million guilders is calculated for 1979.

*11. **Some Economic Consequences of Technological Advance in Medical Care: The Case of a New Drug,** Geweke and Weisbrod, 1981.

Using one of the few data bases computerizing complete treatment costs of a large (Medicaid) population, the authors use naturally generated data to construct a retrospective experiment. Reimbursement costs for cimetidine-treated ulcer patients are compared with costs of traditionally treated ulcer patients. Disease severity is controlled by prior reimbursement level. The new drug intervention is found cost-reductive, a limited criterion not measuring effects on well-being.

12. **Cost-Effectiveness of Duodenal Ulcer Treatment,** Culyer and Maynard, 1981.

This study provides an excellent introduction to the economic evaluation of cimetidine. More specifically, it compares the lifetime costs of continued cimetidine treatment and of immediate vagotomy for the appropriate patient. The total cost to society must include the value of a life shortened by surgical mortality, multiplied by its probability of occurrence. (A surgical mortality of 0.5% is adopted by the authors.) The money value of a life must be estimated. Spending over time must be discounted to a present value. The results are strongly influenced by the life-values and discount rates used, and by the scope of costs (institutional or social) considered. The authors conclude that in England, from the point of view of the National Health Service, surgery seems the cheaper alternative, whereas from the community perspective, surgery is more expensive than cimetidine.

1.

von Haunalter G, Chandler VV:

Cost of ulcer disease in the United States.

Stanford Research Institute, Feb. 1977

Between 1968 and 1975 the prevalence of peptic ulcer disease (PUD) increased about 2 to 3% per year, while the rate per 1,000 population also rose according to government data. In 1975, nearly 4 million people in the United States suffered from PUD. The death rate from peptic ulcer, however, has been declining over the past few years, probably because of more extensive health-care programs and improved treatment methods and surgical procedures.

The total cost of treating ulcer patients includes direct costs of medical care (inpatient hospital care, physician and related treatment, drug therapy, nursing home, and other professional services), plus indirect costs of annual earnings lost because of illness and disablement and lifetime earnings lost because of death.

METHODOLOGY

Direct costs for hospital care were derived by using the bottom-up method, which counts only those patients diagnosed as having ulcers and multiplies by estimated daily charges, taking into consideration hospital size and surgery or lack thereof.

Indirect costs were calculated using annual and lifetime earnings applied to productivity losses and deaths, respectively. This involves a number of assumptions concerning labor-force participation, unemployment rates, value of housewives' services, and other factors.

DIRECT COSTS

Inpatient Hospital Care

Since hospital charges vary according to size, the estimated number of patient days for each hospitalization for a primary diagnosis of ulcer disease was divided into type of hospital (greater than or less than 100 beds) and surgical or nonsurgical days. Hospital charges include board, drugs, use of operating room, staff doctor care, x-rays, and other normal services.

Charges for inpatient hospital care rose from $803 million in 1975 to $1,072 million in 1977 (Table 1). The cost of inpatient hospital care for surgical

Table 1

Estimated Cost of Ulcer Inpatient Hospital Care

1975 Hospital size	Total patient days (thousands)	%	Surgical cases Patient days (thousands)	Daily charges	Total charges (millions)	Nonsurgical cases Patient days (thousands)	Daily charges	Total charges (millions)
<100 beds	672	17	356	$175	$ 62	316	$100	$ 32
>100 beds	3,279	83	1,738	275	478	1,541	150	231
Total	3,951	100	2,094	–	$540	1,857	–	$263
	100%		53%			47%		
1977								
<100 beds	618	16	359	$231	$ 83	260	$132	$ 34
>100 beds	3,246	84	1,882	364	685	1,363	198	270
Total	3,864	100	2,241	–	$768	1,623	–	$304
	100%		58%			42%		

Summary of charges	Millions of dollars	
	1975	1977
Surgical cases	$540	$ 768
Nonsurgical cases	263	304
Total	$803	$1,072

patients in 1977 was estimated at $768 million, in contrast to $304 million for nonsurgical cases. Both figures reflect the fact that large hospitals (>100 beds) charge more per patient-day than do small hospitals (<100 beds).

Physician and Related Treatment Costs

Charges for physician and related treatment services included office and hospital visits, laboratory tests, endoscopic and x-ray examinations, and surgeon's fees. Costs for these services rose from an estimated $240 million in 1975 to $283 million in 1977.

Drug Therapy

Antispasmodics/anticholinergics, tranquilizers, and antacids were the most frequently used drugs considered. The ulcer proportion of self-medicated antacid use was arbitrarily assumed to be half the ulcer proportion in the doctor-originated prescriptions and recommendations. The amount spent for ulcer drug therapy in 1977 was $113 million, which represented an increase of $13 million from 1975.

Nursing Homes and Other Professional Services

The nursing home costs attributable to ulcer disease were estimated at $11 million in 1975 and $15 million in 1977. Other professional services, which consisted of self-employed professionals such as visiting nurses and dietitians, cost an estimated $3 million annually in both 1975 and 1977.

INDIRECT COSTS

Mortality

The present value of lifetime earnings was used to derive mortality costs, which include the value of marketplace earnings and the value of household earnings for women who are primarily housewives. Even though the number of deaths caused by PUD as well as the rate per population has been decreasing in recent years, the mortality costs rose from an estimated $357 million in 1975 to $408 million in 1977.

Table 2

Estimated National Costs and Lost Earnings Due to Ulcer

	Millions of Dollars
Direct costs	1977
Hospital care	$1,072
Physicians & related	283
Drug therapy	113
Nursing home	15
Other professional	3
Total	$1,486
Indirect costs	
Mortality*	408
Morbidity	1,330
Total	$1,738
Grand total	$3,224

*Loss based on lifetime earnings; if losses are calculated only for one year, they amount to $37 million in $1975 and $39 million in 1977.

Morbidity

Morbidity costs were divided into earnings losses suffered by normally productive ulcer patients who had lost workdays due to ulcer, and those patients who are disabled by ulcer disease and unable to work. Normally productive ulcer patients lost an estimated total of $545 million in earnings or service value in 1975 and $650 million in 1977. Losses due to disability rose from an estimated $571 million in 1975 to $680 million in 1977.

CONCLUSION

Direct costs account for slightly less than half the total costs of PUD, but are increasing faster than the other cost components, most likely because the costs of medical care are rising faster than earnings. The largest single cost is due to morbidity, with hospital care being the second largest, and the more rapidly rising, cost. Projected costs in 1977 total $3.2 billion, as summarized in Table 2.

Robinson Associates, Inc:
The impact of cimetidine on the national cost of duodenal ulcers.
Robinson Associates, May, 1978

Since cimetidine was expected to have both direct and indirect impact on national health care costs associated with peptic ulcer disease (PUD) in the United States, a marketing and management consulting firm undertook a study to develop a cost-benefit analysis of the use of cimetidine.

METHODOLOGY

Twenty-three leading independent investigators, who were responsible for the clinical evaluation of cimetidine that was submitted to the FDA, were individually interviewed to develop expected patterns of treatment and response with conventional therapy as well as with cimetidine. The investigators were given descriptions of five paradigmatic cases that covered the spectrum of duodenal ulcer (DU) disease, from mild to severe with bleeding. Each investigator was asked 1) what proportion of the current doctor-treated DU population was represented by each type, 2) how a typical physician would most likely treat each of these patients prior to the introduction of cimetidine, and 3) how he would treat them if he were to prescribe cimetidine, including all drug regimens and dietary changes. The physicians were then asked to estimate how the treatment program would affect the frequency of repeat episodes, patient visits to physicians, hospitalizations, x-ray and endoscopic examinations, the amount of missed work, the likelihood of surgery, and the likelihood of death from ulcer complications. Questions about costs of therapy were *not* asked. Each investigator was further asked to estimate the probability with which other practicing physicians and specialists would prescribe cimetidine and other antiulcer drugs for each of the five types of patients.

These projections were then used along with average charge figures to develop national cost estimates. It was assumed that cimetidine would be administered to 80, 50, or 25% of all ulcer patients, 80% being, in fact, the overall estimate, by the physician panel, of the average projected extent of administration. Included in the cost analysis were the opportunity losses associated with missed work, disability, and death. The estimated percentage cost changes were then applied category by category to the actual costs of DU incurred in the United States during 1977, as projected by the Stanford Research Institute (SRI) study, *Costs of Ulcer Disease in the United States* (February 1977).

GENERAL BACKGROUND COSTS WITHOUT CIMETIDINE

The national ulcer costs in the United States can be separated into direct and indirect costs. Annual costs for gastric and duodenal ulcers for 1977 as projected by SRI are displayed in Table 1. Hospital care is by far the largest component of direct costs, and any percentage savings in this area will dominate any other cost effect resulting from cimetidine. Among the indirect costs, morbidity plays the dominant role. While direct costs are hard

Table 1

Comparison of 1977 Gastric and
Duodenal Ulcer Health Care Costs (in millions)

	Ulcer type		
Cost factor	**Gastric**	**Duodenal**	**Total peptic ulcer**
Direct costs			
Hospital care	$ 340	$ 732	$ 1,072
Physican & related			
MD office/hospital visits:	19	46	65
Laboratory tests	5	9	14
Endoscopic exams	4	7	11
X-Ray exams	28	50	78
Surgeons fees	41	74	115
Drug therapy	28	85	113
Nursing home	4	11	15
Other professional	1	2	3
Total direct costs	$470	$1,016	$1,486
Indirect costs			
Mortality	163	245	408
Morbidity			
Absenteeism	195	455	650
Disability	204	476	680
Total indirect costs	562	1,176	1,738
Grand total	$1,032	$2,192	$3,224

National Costs of Duodenal Ulcers (in Millions), Computed for Various Levels of

Level of Cimetidine Usage

Cost component	Traditional therapy 0%		25%		50%	
	DU Costs($)	Reduction (%)$	DU Costs($)	Reduction (%)($)	DU Costs($)	Reduction (%)($)
Direct costs						
Hospital care	732	0 (0%)	651	81 (11%)	571	161 (22%)
Physicians & Related						
MD office/hospital visits	46	0 (0%)	43	3 (6%)	41	5 (12%)
Laboratory tests	9	– (0%)	9	– (0%)	9	– (0%)
Endoscopic exams	7	0 (0%)	7	50 (6%)	6	1 (13%)
X-ray exam	50	0 (0%)	47	3 (5%)	45	5 (10%)
Surgeons fees	74	0 (0%)	65	9 (-13%)	55	19 (-25%)
Drug therapy	85	0 (0%)	96	-11 (-13%)	106	-21 (-25%)
Nursing home	11	– (0%)	11	– (0%)	11	– (0%)
Other professional	2	– (0%)	2	– (0%)	2	– (0%)
Total direct costs	1,016	0 (0%)	931	85 (8%)	846	170 (17%)
Indirect costs						
Mortality	245	0 (0%)	231	14 (6%)	218	27 (11%)
Morbidity	931	0 (0%)	826	105 (11%)	725	206 (22%)
Absenteeism	455	0 (0%)	407	46 (10%)	362	93 (20%)
Long term disability	476	0 (0%)	419	57 (12%)	363	113 (24%)
Total indirect costs	1,176	0 (0%)	1,057	119 (10%)	943	233 (20%)
Grand total	2,192	0 (0%)	1,990	202 (9%)	1,789	403 (18%)

costs, indirect costs represent lost opportunity costs, which appear in the aggregate national economic statistics such as GNP and a decreased tax base.

FINDINGS: COSTS WITH USE OF CIMETIDINE

The major results of this study indicate that in 1977 a projected 80% usage of cimetidine would have reduced national health care costs associated with DU by $645 million—a 29% reduction (Table 2).

Hospital Costs

Disaggregation of this result shows that the largest predicted reduction in direct costs was in hospital care ($258 million, a 35% reduction over actual costs). Contributing to the decreased hospital costs was a decline in the percent of ulcer patients requiring hospitalization from 31 to 24%. With maximal use of cimetidine, the average hospital stay for the nonsurgical patient declined from 8.6 to 6.2 days. The frequency of readmission declined and the proportion of patients requiring surgery was reduced from 15 to 10%—a 33% reduction overall with maximal (100%) use of cimetidine.

Physician Office/Hospital Visits

Costs for physician office/ hospital visits declined by $8 million (18%) at the 80% utilization rate for

Cimetidine Usage for Year 1977

Predicted level 80%		Predicted level 100%	
DU Costs($)	**Reduction (%)($)**	**DU Costs($)**	**Reduction (%)($)**
474	258 (35%)	435	297 (41%)
38	8 (18%)	37	9 (21%)
9	– (0%)	9	– (0%)
6	1 (20%)	5	2 (24%)
42	8 (16%)	40	10 (20%)
44	30 (41%)	40	34 (46%)
119	-34 (-40%)	128	43 (-50%)
11	– (0%)	11	– (0%)
2	– (0%)	2	– (0%)
745	271 (27%)	707	309 (30%)
201	44 (18%)	196	49 (20%)
602	329 (35%)	548	383 (41%)
307	148 (33%)	277	178 (39%)
295	181 (38%)	271	205 (43%)
803	373 (32%)	744	432 (37%)
1,547	645 (29%)	1,452	740 (34%)

cimetidine because of a significantly diminished need for a doctor to monitor the patient's course during an ulcer attack. It was conservatively assumed that no change occurred in the frequency of attacks with use of cimetidine.

Laboratory Tests, X-rays, and Endoscopies

Although costs for laboratory tests remained the same, costs for x-ray and endoscopic examinations were reduced with 80% cimetidine usage by $8 million (16%) and $1 million (20%), respectively.

Surgeon's Fees

Surgeon's fees were estimated to decline by $30 million, a 41% reduction based on 80% patient usage of cimetidine. This was the largest percentage decrease; it was explained subjectively that one of cimetidine's major benefits was to make surgery unnecessary except in very severe cases involving bleeding or perforation. The percentage of those hospitalized patients who require surgery was expected to drop by one third with the greatest reduction in severe, previously intractable disease.

Mortality

On the average, it was predicted that mortality costs for DU would be reduced by $44 million (18%) with 80% cimetidine usage. Since major risk with DU is the likelihood of surgical complication and since cimetidine significantly lowers the likelihood of surgery, the physician panel generally felt that cimetidine would have its greatest impact on the more severely ill ulcer patients, significantly lowering their need for surgical intervention.

Morbidity

The estimated reduction in indirect costs from absenteeism and long-term disability amounted to $148 million, a 33% reduction and $181 million, a 38% decline, respectively.

Drug Costs

The only category with an increase in costs was the drug category. Estimated drug costs would rise $34 million or 40% predicated on the 80% prescription rate for cimetidine. The physicians interviewed felt that antacids would be used concomitantly with cimetidine but that the use of tranquilizers and anticholinergics would be very low.

DISCUSSION

Based on a collective estimate by leading independent gastroenterological investigators, this study suggests that the national health care costs associated with DU disease will be reduced considerably by the administration of cimetidine. The savings will be implemented through cimetidine's reduction of the severity and duration of DU attacks, leading to major reductions in hospitalization, surgery, and morbidity.

An analysis of individual physician-investigator responses showed variations with respect to the magnitude of changes due to cimetidine therapy. However, the direction of these changes was on the whole consistent, resulting in a net dollar saving with 19 of 23 respondents.

Though it clearly accompanies this saving, the intangible benefit to patients of reduced pain and suffering has not been included in the study.

Ricardo-Campbell R, Eisman MM, Wardell WM, Crossley R:
Preliminary methodology for controlled cost-benefit study of drug impact: The effect of cimetidine on days of work lost in a short-term trial in duodenal ulcer.
Journal of Clinical Gastroenterology 2:37–41, 1980

The productive cost-benefit analysis of a specific therapeutic drug regimen could offer an economic measure of its overall efficacy by indicating its ability to return patients to work. This measure may offer a measure comparable to the traditional clinical one of "global efficacy." The authors proposed to analyze the entity "time lost from work" for duodenal ulcer patients on either cimetidine treatment or on placebo and to examine the results in the two groups for statistically significant differences.

EXPERIMENTAL METHOD

A subset of 64 patients were included in the analysis, out of a potential 217 patients undergoing phase II/III clinical trials. The trials were random and double-blind with patient assignment to either cimetidine and antacid or to placebo and antacid. All patients in the trials had endoscopically proven duodenal ulcers and had ulcer symptoms for at least 3 of the 7 days prior to entering the study. Patients in the subset had lost some time from work during that period. At the end of week 1, 2, 4, and 6 each patient was interviewed and the datum "time lost from work due to ulcer disease during the previous week" was obtained. The subset of workers was small primarily because 47 of the original 217 patients were unemployed and the status of a further 80 was ambiguous.

RESULTS

The improvement during drug treatment as measured by a decline in the quantifiable entity "time lost from work" was significantly greater with cimetidine than it was with placebo. The onset of the cimetidine effect was early, rapid, and evident by the end of the first week of therapy. The weekly decline in absenteeism was consistently greater for the cimetidine group than for the placebo; the difference grew greater each week, and reached a maximum during the last week of the experiment. See the Figure.

Two other noteworthy results were obtained. First, absenteeism from duodenal ulcer disease is distinctly an all or nothing event with most patients either going in to work or staying out for the whole work week. Second, the correlation between the responses to the clinical global measure "overall general feeling" and the actual degree of attendance at work was not statistically significant.

DISCUSSION

Economic cost-benefit analysis in medicine must include the direct medical costs of treatment and the indirect costs that result from lost work and disability. In order to evaluate the indirect costs accurately, the monetary value of an hour's work customarily performed by the patient is desirable.

This study strongly suggests that cimetidine returns patients to their employment sooner than does placebo, but because of uncertainty about the value of the work performed by the subjects in this

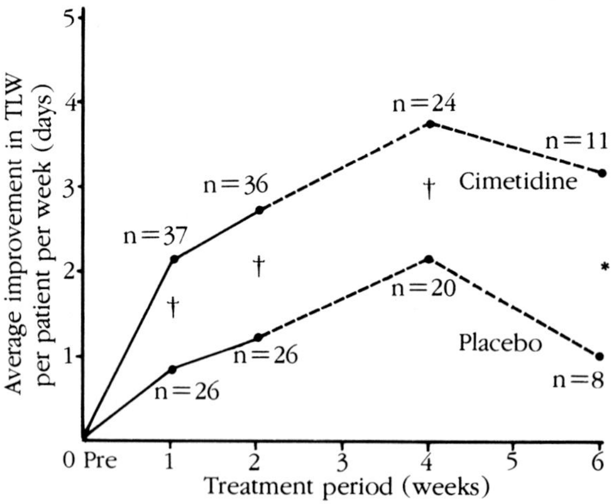

Figure. Improvement in TLW (time lost from work during the previous week because of ulcer disease) as a function of duration of treatment in cimetidine- and placebo-treated groups, using pooled data. Improvement with cimetidine treatment at weeks 1, 2, 4, and 6 was significantly greater than with placebo treatment (*<0.05, †<0.01). The solid line connecting data points at pre-, 1, and 2 weeks indicates that data from these weeks were common to all three studies (ie, 2-, 4-, and 6-weeks). In contrast, data from weeks 4 and 6 were not common to all three studies; hence, a broken line connects the data points at weeks 4 and 6.

study a monetary amount could not be calculated. Improvements in the accuracy of the study could have been obtained if the employment status of everyone in the patient population had been estimated by the clinical investigators.

This study is a pilot study performed in the context of phase II/III clinical trials to test the feasibility of this type of research. The authors conclude that the vehicle is a good one and that this kind of prospective economic analysis is essential to the full recognition of all costs and benefits. According to this philosophy, a quality of life analysis by means of psychological or sociological techniques could also be conducted and evaluated at the same time. Properly designed, such an approach could add valuable new data bases with which to assess the costs and benefits of drug therapy.

4.

Bodemar G, Walan A:
Maintenance treatment of recurrent peptic ulcer by cimetidine.
Lancet 1:403–407, 1978

A 1-year, double-blind trial that assessed the efficacy and safety of cimetidine compared to placebo in chronic peptic ulcers clearly demonstrated that a 1-year maintenance treatment with cimetidine prevents both recurrence and complications of peptic ulcers. Cimetidine significantly reduced work absenteeism, antacid consumption, ulcer pain, and frequency of other symptoms. The only probable side effect of cimetidine was reversible drug-induced liver damage of hypersensitivity type in one patient.

PATIENTS AND METHODS

Adults with proven recurrent ulcers (68), either duodenal (42), peptic (17), or gastric (9), were included in the trial. Patients entered the trial only when endoscopy revealed no ulcers (65 patients had been treated previously with cimetidine) in patients who had previously suffered from ulcers. The cimetidine group, randomly allocated to maintenance treatment for up to 1 year on 400 mg twice daily, consisted of 32 patients: 4 women and 28 men with a mean age of 50.7 years (range 32–67 years); the mean duration of illness was 13.6 years. The group receiving placebo consisted of 36 patients: 6 women and 30 men with a mean age of 50.1 years and 10.7 years of illness.

The patients were followed monthly, and such data as severity of pain, antacid consumption, general well-being, and number of days absent from work because of ulcers were measured. A standard pentagastrin test was performed before the trial, during the fifth week of any recurrence, after 7 months on maintenance treatment, immediately before the end of the trial, and after completion of long-term treatment. Standard laboratory and statistical measuring methods were used.

If an ulcer developed, open treatment with cimetidine 1 g daily was given until complete healing (by endoscopy); then patients returned to their original maintenance treatment.

RESULTS

Endoscopy Findings
Six of 32 patients on cimetidine had endoscopically proven recurrent ulcers compared to 30 of 36 patients on placebo. No patients in the cimetidine group had complications while four in the placebo group did (three requiring hospitalization). One of 32 patients on cimetidine, compared to 15 on placebo, needed surgery because they had two recurrences or because of severe symptoms at the first recurrence. The results are summarized in the Table. Only 20% of the cimetidine group, compared to 45% of the placebo group, still had moderate or severe duodenitis and gastritis after 7 and 12 months of treatment.

Symptoms
The cimetidine group (20 of 32) had a significant reduction in the incidence of both day and night pain when compared to the placebo group (6 of 36). Antacid consumption was also significantly lower in the cimetidine group, and the patients' overall assessment of their general well-being was

Table

Clinical Outcome of Trial

	Cimetidine (n=32)	Placebo (n=36)
Total	6	30
Duodenal ulcer	3 (n=19)	18 (n=23)
Pyloric ulcer	3 (n=8)	8 (n=9)
Gastric ulcer	0 (n=5)	4 (n=4)
No. with 2 recurrences	1	12
No. with complications	0	4
No. operated on	1	15

n = no. of patients in the group

significantly better. One of the 32 patients on cimetidine was off work for 79 days because of symptoms, while 23 of the 36 patients on placebo were off work for a total of 1,405 days (mean of 2.8 days per patient per year on cimetidine compared to 49.3 days on placebo).

Other Findings

Acid secretion and blood levels of cimetidine patients remained even during the year, with no evidence of rebound effect either 2 days or 3 1/2 months after stopping long-term treatment. None of the cimetidine-treated patients had any complications in the 6 months after the end of the trial.

The few patients in the cimetidine group who had a relapse during the trial were healed within 6 weeks by an increased dose of cimetidine. When patients with severe symptoms had to be given therapeutic doses, symptoms disappeared within 1 week in 50% having their first course, in 57% having their second course, and in 50% having their third course of 1 g of cimetidine daily.

Side Effects

Isolated instances of mental confusion, muscle twitches in a patient with renal failure, and exacerbation of ileus in burn cases possibly related to cimetidine treatment have been reported elsewhere. Gynecomastia and galactorrhea can develop. In this study, the only probable and serious side effect was reversible liver damage of the hypersensitive type in 1 patient. The rise (to within normal limits) of serum creatinine at the start of treatment with cimetidine still needs to be explained. There were no abnormal hematological values in these patients on long-term treatment with cimetidine. The drug seems still to be reasonably safe.

REFERENCES

1. Stanford Research Institute: *Cost of Ulcer Disease in the United States.* Philadelphia, Smith Kline & French Corporation, 1977
2. Netherlands Economic Institute: *Present Cost of Peptic Ulceration to the Dutch Economy and Possible Impact of Cimetidine on This Cost.* Holland, Smith Kline & French, 1977
3. Institute of Political Economic Studies, University of Pavia: *The Determination of the Social Costs of Peptic Ulcer in Italy.* Italy, Smith Kline & French Corporation, 1978
4. Hertzman P, Jönsson B: *Magsårssjukdomens Sambälls-ekonomiska Kostnader.* The Swedish Institute for Health Economics, Lund, 1977
5. Bodemar G, Walan A: Two-year follow-up after one year's treatment with cimetidine or placebo. *Lancet* 1:38, 1980

5.

Bodemar G, Gotthard R, Ström M, Walan A, Jönsson B, Bjurulf P:
Socioeconomic aspects of treatment with cimetidine in peptic ulcer disease, in *Further Experience with H$_2$-Receptor Antagonists in Peptic Ulcer Disease and Progress in Histamine Research.*
Proceedings of the Symposium held at Capri, October 18–20, 1979. Amsterdam, Excerpta Medica

SOCIOECONOMIC COSTS OF PEPTIC ULCER DISEASE

Peptic ulcer disease (PUD) afflicts 10–15% of adult men and 4–15% of adult women in the Western world at least once during their lives. Because the disease is chronic and primarily affects people during their most productive years, its cost to society can be high. The costs involved are *direct* (cost of hospitalization and surgery, physician care and diagnostic procedures, and drugs) and *indirect* (loss of productivity due to absenteeism and mortality resulting from the disease).

Studies have reported the costs of peptic ulcers in the United States, The Netherlands, Italy, and Sweden. The direct costs were highest in the

United States. In Sweden, a decline in hospitalization was due to a tendency not to hospitalize peptic ulcer patients undergoing medical treatment. Before the introduction of cimetidine, the United States spent most of its drug costs on antacids and anticholinergics.

In the United States, The Netherlands, and Sweden, peptic ulcer symptoms caused 1.5% of all days off due to illness. In 1975, it cost the United States $1,330 million (8.6 million working days); in 1977, about 80,000 ulcer patients were chronically disabled. These figures do not consider the decreased capacity of the patients who remain at work; although this cannot be calculated, it probably is an important factor. The average time off in the United States for ulcer patients was 12 (27 in severe cases) compared with 35 days in Italy and 45 in The Netherlands. About 20% of the patients with active ulcers in The Netherlands were absent for more than 3 months, and surgical patients for an average of 3 months; in Sweden, patients in the 25-44 year age group were off work for an average of 4 weeks, in the 45–54 year age group for 6 weeks, and older patients for about 5 weeks—the number of weeks absent had increased since 1963. The costs of peptic ulcer disease are shown in Table 1.

ESTIMATED CHANGES IN SOCIO-ECONOMIC COSTS CAUSED BY CIMETIDINE TREATMENT

Treatment of PUD with cimetidine may decrease the costs of this disease to society. Table 2 suggests potential decreases with cimetidine therapy as estimated by clinicians, assuming a lesser need for hospitalization and a smaller loss of productivity due to decreased absenteeism. These have never been studied in a double-blind trial.

Table 1

The Cost of Peptic Ulcer Disease Before the Introduction of Cimetidine Therapy

	U.S.A.[1] (1977) 3,224 million dollars		The Netherlands[2] (1975) 337 million guilders		Italy[3] (1976) 284 billion lire		Sweden[4] (1975) 480 million croner	
Total cost								
Direct costs (%)	46		21		42		22	
Hospital care		33		18		24		15
Physician care		9		2		7		4
Drugs		4		1		11		3
Indirect costs	54		79		58		78	
Absenteeism		41		79		58		68
Mortality*		13		0		0		10
Total (%)	100	100	100	100	100	100	100	100

*Calculated with discounts of 2.5% for the U.S.A. and 6% for Sweden; the U.S.A. estimate assumes a 2% increase in productivity and 6% inflation.

Table 2

Clinicians' Assumptions of Cost Benefit of Cimetidine, Expressed as Percentages of the Total Costs

	U.S.A.		The Netherlands	Italy
Cimetidine usage (%)	**50**	**80**	**50**	**100**
Direct costs (%)	17	27	20	19
Hospital care	22	35	28	66
Physician care	12	18	0	0
Drugs	-25	-40	-91	-101
Indirect costs (%)	20	32	21	40
Absenteeism	22	35	21	40
Mortality	11	18	0	0
Total savings (%)	18	29	21	31

Table 3

Clinical Outcome During and 2 Years After the Trial

	Placebo group (n=35[*])	Cimetidine (n=31[†])
During trial		
Referred for surgery	15	1
Bleeding ulcers	4	0
After trial		
Months after end of trial with mild or no symptoms mean and (range)	8.8 (1–22)	10.1 (0.5–24)
Referred for surgery	7	2
Bleeding ulcers	1	1
Not operated	13	27
No symptoms[†]	4	8
Mild symptoms[‡]	2	8
Moderate symptoms[§]	7	8
Severe symptoms[‖]	0	3

*One patient stopped treatment during the trial because of myocardial infarction; the patient with bleeding ulcer after the trial is included in the patients who were operated on. †One patient stopped treatment during the trial because of cardiac failure; the patient with bleeding ulcer after the trial, who refused surgery, is included in the 8 patients with moderate symptoms. ‡No cimetidine administered after the maintenance trial; §short courses of cimetidine administered after trial; ‖cimetidine administered almost continuously after the trial.

ABSENTEEISM BEFORE AND DURING MAINTENANCE TREATMENT WITH CIMETIDINE

A previous study reported the results of a double-blind, long-term maintenance trial in 68 patients with chronic ulcers. Many of these patients had taken increasing time from work due to illness in the preceding 3 years. Most patients had received 1 g/day of cimetidine, and the ulcers were healed within 2 weeks. For the next year 32 patients were maintained on 400 mg cimetidine twice daily and 36 received a placebo, also given twice daily. When recurrence occurred, open cimetidine 1 g/day was given for 6 weeks; then patients were either readmitted to double-blind maintenance or underwent surgery. All patients were allowed antacid tablets for relief of symptoms during the trial.

The results of the 1-year maintenance were as follows: In the cimetidine group five patients had one recurrence, one had two recurrences, none had complications, and one was operated on; in the placebo group, 18 patients had 1 recurrence, 12 had 2 recurrences (4 with complications), and 15 were operated on. All recurrences were determined by endoscopy.

An important finding is the number of patients maintained on cimetidine who were absent from work during the 1-year trial period: only 1 patient in this group needed to be absent from work during the course of the trial, compared with 15 in the preceding year. Treatment with placebo, however, did not change the number of patients who needed time off: of the 36 patients maintained on placebo, 24 had been absent from work during the year preceding the trial and 23, with endoscopically proven re-ulceration, were absent for varying lengths of time during the maintenance period.

RECURRENCE OF PEPTIC ULCER AFTER CIMETIDINE

Cimetidine promotes healing and prevents the recurrence of ulcers. But what happens after cimetidine treatment is reduced? In a previously reported study, 60 patients whose ulcers had healed with cimetidine, placebo, or antacid-anticholinergics were followed up for 1 year after the discontinuation of therapy. Since the number of patients whose ulcers healed on each of the two active regimens did not differ statistically, a difference in relapse rates after discontinuation of treatment would indicate whether either regimen itself influenced relapse after discontinuation. Twelve of 20 cimetidine-treated patients had a relapse after median time of 2.5 months, and 9 of 20 patients treated with the antacid-anticholinergic combination had recurring ulcers after 4 months. These differences were not statistically significant.

Cimetidine was more effective than the antacid-anticholinergic combination in relieving pain. It is possible that the cimetidine-treated patients changed their life-style—increased alcohol intake, work hours, etc—to the degree where they would have to stay on the drug to remain symptom-free. Once treatment stops, these etiologic factors must be dealt with to prevent reaggravation of the ulcers.

RECURRENCE OF ULCERS 2 YEARS AFTER CIMETIDINE MAINTENANCE TREATMENT

What happens after long-term treatment is stopped? Patients in the 1-year maintenance study were followed up for 2 years after the trial's conclusion. The results suggest that the severity of chronic PUD is favorably influenced by 1 year's treatment with cimetidine and that this influence continues even after treatment is stopped. When moderate or severe symptoms developed after trial, they were well controlled by short courses of treatment with cimetidine or, in three patients, with almost continuous treatment. The entire 3-year period is summarized in Table 3. One noteworthy statistic is that of the 32 patients from the cimetidine group, 7 were or should have been operated on, compared with 22 of the 36 patients from the placebo group.

FUTURE ASPECTS

A Swiss study suggests that for PUD the least expensive treatment, as compared to selective proximal vagotomy, is administration of a nightly dose of cimetidine for 15 years, operating only on patients who have a recurrence more than twice during that period. This finding is based on the cost of postsurgical syndromes, including chronic disability, which was three times higher than the initial cost of surgery. A Danish study has shown that the majority of patients probably do not need 15 years of treatment before ulcers cease to be active.

Cimetidine reduces the need for surgery during treatment. If this reduction can also be achieved after therapy is stopped, it would substantially add to the already great economic benefits offered by this drug. The results of long-term toxicity studies will tell decisively whether or not long-term cimetidine treatment can be undertaken.

Reprinted with permission. H_2 Receptor Antagonists in Peptic Ulcer Disease and Progress in Histamine Research, European Symposium, Capri, 1979. ICS 521, Excerpta Medica—Amsterdam.

6.

Fineberg HV, Pearlman LA:
Surgical treatment of peptic ulcer in the United States: Trends before and after the introduction of cimetidine.
Lancet 1:1305–1307, 1981

Peptic ulcers affect millions of Americans at some point in their lives. Somewhat less than 250,000 Americans develop new peptic ulcers each year; new duodenal ulcers are more than four times as common as new gastric ulcers.

The number of operations for peptic ulcer fell significantly further in 1978 than expected, and the greater number of operations in 1979 was still significantly below that predicted by the trend from 1966 to 1977, but not below that predicted by the figures from 1973 to 1977.

In August, 1977, the FDA approved cimetidine for up to 8 weeks' use in patients with duodenal ulcers and hypersecretory conditions. By 1978, the National Disease and Therapeutic Index recorded that 3 million patients with ulcer disease had been treated with the drug. Gastroenterological problems other than peptic ulcer now account for more than 50% of the drug's use. This study examined the ulcer statistics to see if there was a correlation between increased use of cimetidine and fewer surgical procedures for ulcers.

METHODS

The Hospital Discharge Survey of the U.S. National Center for Health Statistics (NCHS) samples from the population of all nonfederal, short-term hospitals, stratified by size and location, and then projects these results into national statistics. These statistics were used to work out the pattern of ulcer surgery before and after the introduction of cimetidine.

RESULTS

The principal operations for ulcer disease are partial gastrectomy and vagotomy. Nearly all vagotomies since 1966 were probably for ulcer disease; most partial gastrectomies were performed for ulcer disease as well. In 1966, 136,000 of these operations were performed in the United States; by 1977, this had fallen to 97,000, almost a 30% decline.

In 1978, the first whole year after cimetidine's introduction, the number of operations dropped to 69,000. Although the number rose to 81,000 in 1979, it is still significantly below the rates predicted on the basis of the trend from 1966 to 1977 (Figure 1). The number of operations in 1979 was well within the 95% confidence interval of the linear regression line for 1973 to 1977 (Figure 2). Moreover, the proportion of hospital admissions for ulcer disease was between 25 and 29% from 1966 to 1979; in 1978, the figure was 19%. In the decade before 1978, therefore, one in four patients admitted to the hospital for peptic ulcers was operated upon, while in 1978 the number dropped to below one in five.

DISCUSSION

Compared with other abdominal operations, surgery for ulcer disease shows a striking drop in 1978 (Table). This striking decline could be the result of

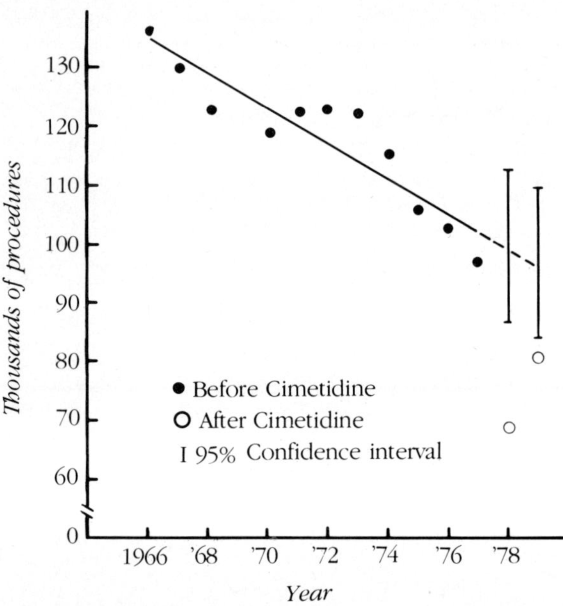

Figure 1. Partial gastrectomy and vagotomy surgery in the United States, 1966–79.

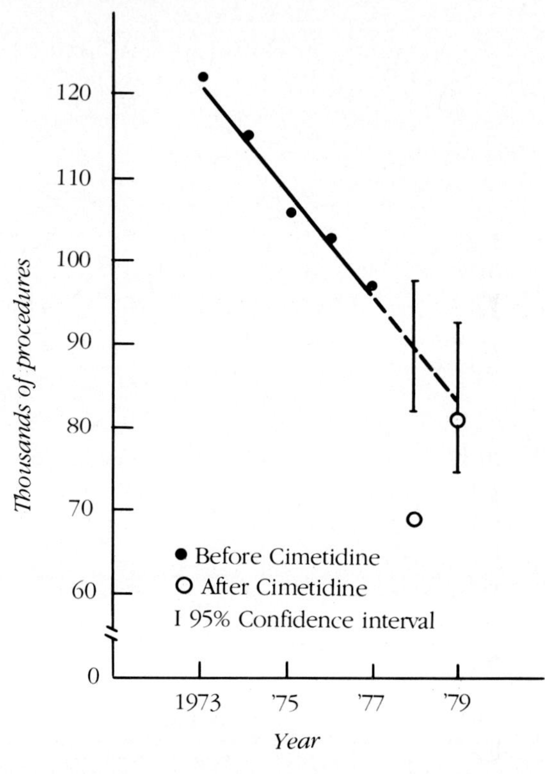

Figure 2. Partial gastrectomy and vagotomy surgery in the United States, 1973–79.

Table

Selected Abdominal Surgical Procedures: Rate per 10,000 Population

Procedure	1970	1975	1976	1978
All abdominal surgery	122	138	133	132
Partial gastrectomy and vagotomy	6	5	5	3
Appendicectomy	16	15	14	14
Cholecystectomy	18	21	21	20
Herniorrhaphy	25	26	24	24

Source: National Center for Health Statistics, National Hospital Discharge Survey

a more cautious attitude toward operations in general, especially elective ones. No comparable decline is noted, however, for herniorrhaphy, which is more often an elective procedure than is surgery for ulcer disease. Diagnostic advances seem unlikely to have caused such a precipitous decline in 1978.

The efficacy of cimetidine in promoting the healing of duodenal ulcer is well documented as is its ability to reduce the risk of recurrence during maintenance treatment for as long as 1 year. The fact that surgery is often delayed while a patient is on cimetidine may account for the rise in operations in 1979, since those patients who were not operated on in 1978 may have undergone surgery in 1979. This, however, cannot be verified by available data.

The extensive use and efficacy of cimetidine may account for the unexpectedly large decline in surgery in 1978. Corroborative evidence could come from similar patterns in other countries and from studies testing the association between absence of cimetidine treatment and ulcer surgery.

7.

Wyllie JH, Williams JA, Kennedy TL, Clark CG, Bell PRF, Kirk RM, MacKay C:
Effect of cimetidine on surgery for duodenal ulcer.
Lancet 1:1307–1308, 1981

Much has been written about the effectiveness of cimetidine in clinical trials. It does not tell us whether the drug, when freely prescribed, proves useful. For example, does cimetidine reduce the need for ulcer surgery?

METHODS

To determine the effect of cimetidine on the frequency of surgery for duodenal ulcer, information from 6 hospitals in Great Britain engaged in the surgical treatment of duodenal ulcers was compared on the basis of the number of operations performed for 5 years before and 4 years after the introduction of cimetidine in November, 1976.

Information was collected on the number of operations performed per year for duodenal ulcers. Both emergency and elective operations were included since there is often no clear distinction between them. Furthermore, no differentiation was made between primary operations and those to treat ulcers that had recurred after previous surgery.

RESULTS

The overall results are shown in the Figure. From 1972 to 1976, the number of operations averaged 477 per year and since then has fallen to 290 per year, a reduction of 39.2%. Results by hospital are in the Table.

DISCUSSION

The number of operations performed from 1977 to 1980 was markedly less than expected. The change in surgical practice from a total of 461 operations in 1976 to 283 in 1977, coincident with the

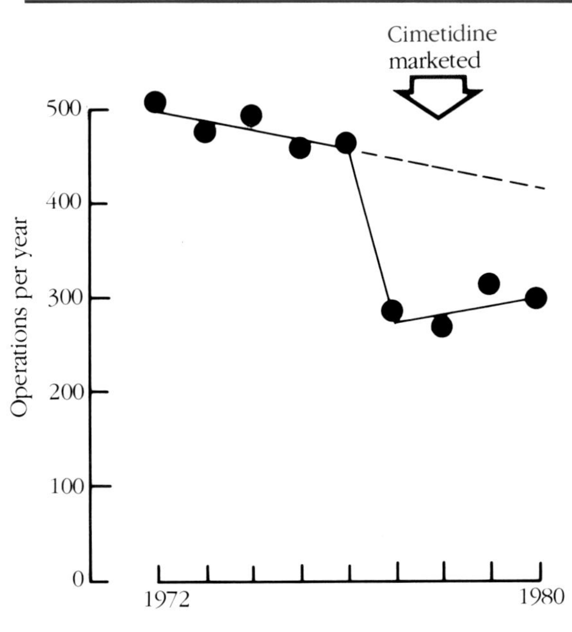

Figure. Operations for duodenal ulceration each year from 1972 to 1980.

Table

Number of Operations Performed Annually for Duodenal Ulceration From 1972–1980

| Center | 1972 | Before cimetidine | | | | After cimetidine | | | | Center totals | Expected (no./yr) | 1972–80 χ^2 with 8df | |
		1973	1974	1975	1976	1977	1978	1979	1980			χ^2	P
1	84	99	112	126	99	97	79	118	112	926	102.9	18.7	<0.05
2	133	115	126	110	125	72	80	74	61	896	99.6	61.2	<0.001
3	96	94	99	70	71	32	29	37	27	555	61.7	122.1	<0.001
4	72	63	73	55	79	40	47	37	47	513	57.0	33.2	<0.001
5	75	77	40	58	45	20	5	23	30	373	41.4	119.1	<0.001
6	45	24	42	38	42	22	25	24	23	285	31.7	24.1	<0.01
Totals	505	472	492	457	461	283	265	313	300	3548	394.2	205.0	<0.001

Center 3: a trial of ranitidine was undertaken in 1980 and emergency operations were omitted.
Center 2: gastric, as well as duodenal ulcers were included.

introduction of cimetidine, argues strongly for cause and effect. There was no other major advance in the therapy of duodenal ulcers. The number of operations for duodenal ulcers in Britain has been falling for more than 10 years. The initial impact of cimetidine, however, was a 38.3% drop in surgery. The regression in the yearly number of operations in each center before and after the introduction of cimetidine shows that although the mean slope was reduced from 1977 to 1980, the change was not significant. Thus, there is no evidence that the effect of cimetidine has diminished.

Surgery in ulcer patients is usually recommended when medical treatment has failed. A true test of cimetidine's efficacy would thus be whether the centers that specialize in the treatment of duodenal ulcers have experienced a fall, such as that above in the number of patients referred to them or on whom they felt operation was justified. Such a test seems to provide a better indication of the efficacy of cimetidine in general use than do strictly controlled clinical trials from which patients defect.

8.

Venables CW:

Surgery and hospitalization trends in the UK before and after cimetidine: A talk given at the symposium;
Cimetidine, Surgery Trends and the Cost of Peptic Ulcer Disease, Amsterdam, March 20, 1981 (proceedings in press)

Peptic ulcer is a chronic relapsing disease, which usually lasts for years and often for a lifetime. We need to know whether cimetidine alters the natural history of peptic ulcer and reduces the need for other forms of treatment, particularly surgery, which until now was the only form of treatment suitable for patients with frequent relapse.

THE EFFECT OF CIMETIDINE

At least 40% of ulcer patients may require surgery, since cimetidine will not heal 20% of ulcer initially, and another 20% will not be healed even with long-term therapy. If cimetidine did not alter the natural history of the peptic ulcer disease but, rather, delayed the need for surgery, with time we might expect a rebound effect in operations. In the U.K. nationally the frequency of duodenal ulcer surgery, which already was on a downward trend, experienced a dramatic 49% drop after cimetidine was introduced in 1976 (Figure 1). In fact, the frequency of duodenal ulcer surgery since has plateaued and no rebound has been seen through 1978.

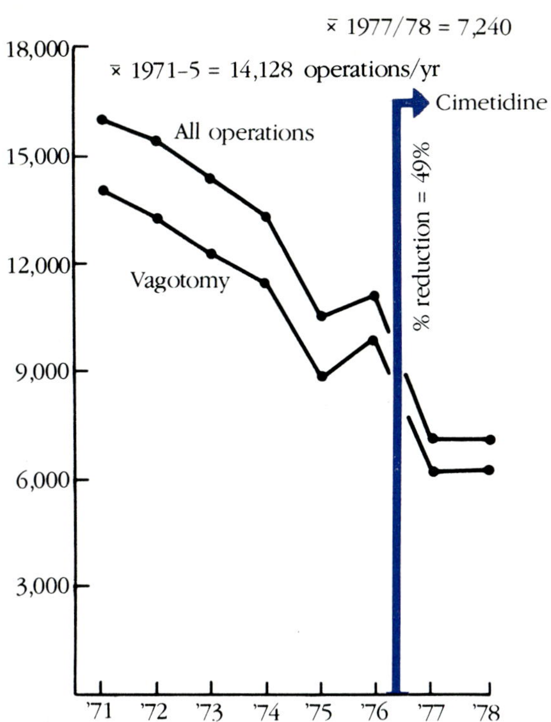

Figure 1. Operation for duodenal ulcer. England & Wales (H.I.P.E.). In 1975 there was an industrial action by junior doctors, which had a marked effect on the number of patients treated in that year.

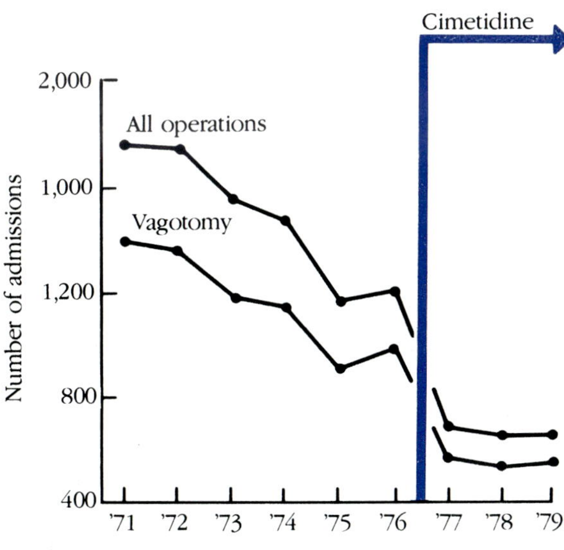

Figure 2. All operations for duodenal ulcer 1971–79 (exluding perforations). Northern region.

Data from the Northern Region of England show the same pattern but through 1979, with no rebound in that year (Figure 2).

Perforation

On the other hand, emergency intestinal perforation, although low in frequency, seems to be related epidemiologically to the incidence of the disease in the community. Cimetidine has not reduced the frequency of this complication in the Northern Region of England, where data are now available. This result suggests that cimetidine, in exerting its therapeutic action, does not affect the basic epidemiology of ulcer disease.

Gastric Ulceration

The frequency of surgery for gastric ulcer, in the U.K. nationally and in the Northern Region, is similar to that of duodenal ulcer: an annual downward trend until the introduction of cimetidine, which signalled the start of a rapid drop over the following 2 years, again, without evidence of a rebound effect.

Long-term

The above suggest that cimetidine is having a long-lasting effect on the need for operation. Whether this will continue depends more on confidence in the drug than upon any other factor, the author believes. Doctors are reluctant to embark upon long-term medical treatments without knowing long-term safety. If doctors remain confident in the safe use of cimetidine, the drop in operations should be maintained.

ECONOMIC IMPLICATION OF MAINTENANCE CIMETIDINE THERAPY

With the cooperation of the author this has been analyzed, using cost data from the Northern Region's Newcastle Royal Victoria Infirmary, by economists AJ Culyer and AK Maynard of York University. Their findings appear in *Social Science and Medicine* (150:8–11, 1981). These authors judge, after due consideration of discount rates and the inadequate basis for calculating the human-capital cost of death from surgery, that long-term drug treatment with cimetidine is substantially less costly than surgery for duodenal ulcer patients.

9.

Rhode Island Health Services Research, Inc:
The effect of cimetidine on peptic ulcer disease in Rhode Island. Submitted as a final report to Smith Kline & French, July 8, 1981

This study evaluated the probable economic costs and benefits of cimetidine as a treatment for peptic ulcer disease and specifically for duodenal ulcers. Both direct and indirect costs to society were studied through evaluation of patterns of hospital use, outpatient treatment, and workdays lost. This survey utilized survey instruments and a large population base. As opposed to controlled clinical trials, such a data base allows extrapolation of empirical findings to a general population.

The following data sources were used: Rhode Island hospital discharge data, to determine any changes in the pattern of hospital use since cimetidine; a Household Interview Survey, to investigate changes in ambulatory treatment (a follow-up was designed for families reporting ulcer disease and permission to recontact them was secured); and the Temporary Disability Insurance (TDI) plan, which provided a data source for investigating changes in work-loss days due to ulcer before and after the introduction of cimetidine.

The study allowed some national data projections based on the Rhode Island experience.

LITERATURE REVIEW AND STUDY OBJECTIVES

The underlying technique in estimating costs of illness is to divide the costs into three types: 1) direct (expenses for a particular illness), 2) indirect (loss of output due to morbidity or premature mortality caused by the illness), and 3) emotional (pain and suffering).

Other studies have projected major direct and indirect cost savings from cimetidine use. What these reports lack, however, are empirical data from the entire population of a specified jurisdiction. The present study provides population-based analysis of hospitalization and associated costs for ulcer patients.

HOSPITALIZATION FOR PEPTIC ULCERS IN RHODE ISLAND

The study linked medical record abstracts and Blue Cross bills to estimate the total effect on charges for hospital services in Rhode Island associated with the introduction of cimetidine. Hospital cases were

selected by the diagnosis stated on the medical record and by the major surgical procedures used to treat ulcers. This evaluated the match between the stated surgical procedure used to treat ulcers and the stated ulcer diagnosis. Rates were taken before and after cimetidine's introduction to the market.

Data Sources and Methods

The medical record data used were the Uniform Hospital Discharge Data Set (UHDDS), which included age, sex, residence, admission and discharge dates, diagnoses, and accompanying surgical procedures, if any. All patients who resided in Rhode Island were included minus those who migrated out of state for care. Billing information came from Rhode Island Blue Cross/Blue Shield and was matched to the medical record. This link allowed the investigators to determine hospital charges for each type of hospitalization studied.

Table 1 shows the rates of hospital discharge for duodenal ulcer during the pre- and post-cimetidine periods of use. No significant change between 1978 and prior year is evident.

Evaluation of Hospital Use by Surgery Data

Surgical data prove more valuable than diagnosis data because they are more accurate and can provide a more detailed evaluation. The surgeries selected were the major ones, partial gastrectomy and vagotomy; this study reviewed the medical literature and found no unanimous procedure of choice among surgeons. A medical or surgical approach often depends on the physician's preference and differs from patient to patient.

Table 2 shows the rates of hospital discharge for partial gastrectomy and/or vagotomy surgery from 1973 through 1979. Note the difference beginning with 1978 when cimetidine had been in use for its first complete year. The number of hospitalizations and discharge rate for operations (without neoplasm) were significantly different. These statistics are also presented graphically in Figure 1, which illustrates that the introduction of cimetidine coincided with a sharp reduction in the number of surgical procedures in ulcer cases. Because there is

Table 1

Hospital Discharges, Ulcer Hospitalizations, Hospital Discharge Rates per 10,000 Persons,
and Average Length of Stay; for Rhode Island Residents for the 12 Months
Ending August 31, 1973 Through 1979

| | **Years ending August 31** | | | | | | |
| | **Pre-test periods** | | | | | **Post-test periods** | |
	1973	**1974**	**1975**	**1976**	**1977**	**1978**	**1979**
Duodenal ulcer							
Number of hospitalizations	901	942	846	721	730	742	627
Discharge rate per 10,000 population	9.5	10.3	9.3	8.0	8.0	8.1	6.9

| | **Observed numbers and rates for years ending August 31** | | | **95% confidence interval and predicted rate for 1978 and 1979 based on 1973–1977 data** | |
	1978	**1979**	**Statistical test**	**1978**	**1979**
Duodenal ulcer					
Number of hospitalizations	742	627			
Discharge rate per 10,000 population	8.1	6.9	Linear regression	7.4±3.0	6.8±3.5
			Natural log transformation with linear regression	7.5+2.9, 7.5–2.1	7.0+3.2, 7.0–2.2

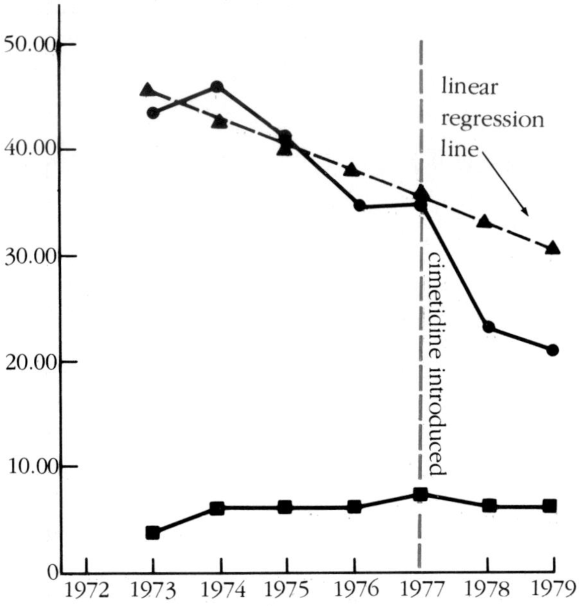

● Ulcer surgery
▲ Linear regression line
■ Neoplasm

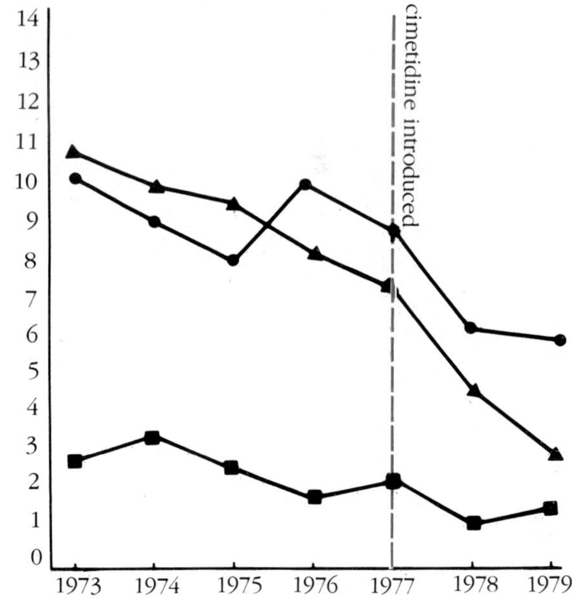

■ 15–44
▲ 45–64
● 65 +

Figure 1. Rates per 100,000 persons for partial gastrectomy and/or vagotomy for Rhode Island residents for the 12 months ending in August 31, 1973 through 1979.

Figure 2. Age specific rates per 10,000 persons for ulcer surgery for Rhode Island residents for the 12 months ending August 31, 1973 through 1979.

Table 2

Hospital Discharges, Hospital Discharge Rates per 10,000 Persons for Partial Gastrectomy and/or Vagotomy for Rhode Island Residents for the 12 Months Ending August 31, 1973 through 1979

	Years ending August 31						
	Pre-test periods					Post-test periods	
	1973	**1974**	**1975**	**1976**	**1977**	**1978**	**1979**
Partial gastrectomy and/or vagotomy *without* a diagnosis of neoplasm							
Number of hospitalizations	412	414	373	331	324	211	192
Discharge rate per 10,000 persons	4.4	4.5	4.1	3.6	3.6	2.3	2.1
Partial gastrectomy and/or vagotomy *with* a diagnosis of neoplasm							
Number of hospitalizations	47	65	67	64	69	66	63
Discharge rate per 10,000 persons	0.5	0.7	0.7	0.7	0.8	0.7	0.7

	Observed numbers and rates for years ending August 31			95% confidence interval and predicted rate for 1978 and 1979 based on 1973-1977 data	
	1978	**1979**	**Statistical test**	**1978**	**1979**
Partial gastrectomy and/or vagotomy *without* a diagnosis of neoplasm					
Number of hospitalizations	211	192			
Discharge rate per 10,000 persons	2.3*†	2.1†	Linear regression	3.3±0.9	3.0±1.0
			Natural log transformation with linear regression	3.3+0.9, 3.3-0.6	3.1+0.8, 3.1-0.7
Partial gastrectomy and/or vagotomy *with* a diagnosis of neoplasm					
Number of hospitalizations	66	63			
Discharge rate per 10,000 persons	0.7	0.7	Critical ratio	0.7±0.3‡	0.7±0.3

*Using linear regression, the change is significant, $p < 0.05$
†Using natural log transformation the linear regression change is significant, $p < 0.05$
‡If the 4 years, 1974 through 1977, are used instead of 1973 through 1977, the mean is 0.7 and the confidence interval is reduced to 0.1. Nevertheless, there is no significant change

no subsequent increase in ulcer surgery in 1979, this would suggest that the sudden decline in ulcer surgery in 1978 was not simply due to postponements of ulcer surgery.

The age groups of 45–64 years and 65+ years also declined in surgery rates from what would have been predicted, after the introduction of cimetidine. Figure 2 illustrates the difference in the numbers of surgical procedures for the three age groups used. The Health Interview Survey also found that cimetidine was most frequently prescribed in the 45–64 age group, which showed the most rapid decline in surgery.

Declines in the use of ulcer surgery following the introduction of cimetidine also occur in each of the three geographical areas of Rhode Island.

Other Factors

It is possible that factors other than the introduction of cimetidine could have caused the accelerated statewide decline in surgery in 1978.

(1) Physician manpower characteristics were

analyzed. There was no unusual increase or decrease in the supply or mix of surgeons, internists, or gastroenterologists after the time cimetidine was introduced.

(2) Various types of ulcer surgery were analyzed to see if there was any unusual shift from one type of ulcer surgery to another around the time cimetidine was introduced. No unusual change, such as a move away from partial gastrectomy to selective or parietal cell vagotomy was found.

(3) A review of drug marketing information for Rhode Island reported in Drug Distribution Data showed a notable decline in sales and market share of all antacid products after the introduction of cimetidine.

(4) The possibility of a decrease in the prevalence of ulcer disease was reviewed by using household surveys conducted in 1975 and 1980. The prevalence of ulcer and ulcer-related conditions in the Rhode Island population increased rather than decreased between 1975 and 1980. Therefore, the possibility of a decline in prevalence of ulceration as a possible factor causing the decline in surgery in 1978 should be ruled out.

To recapitulate, it appears that the introduction of cimetidine may have accelerated in Rhode Island the already evident trend toward substitution of medical for surgical management of ulcer disease.

Cost Implications

Blue Cross and Blue Shield charges for hospitalized ulcer patients are shown in Table 3. Cost savings associated with cimetidine-related avoidance of surgery were calculated under two assumptions: 1) cimetidine patients were hospitalized and only costs of surgery were saved; and 2) the surgical patients were not hospitalized at all, and thus costs of both hospitalization and surgery were saved. If cimetidine is viewed as an intervention under the more conservative assumption 1 above, the saving

in hospital charges was $185,076 and the reduction in physician charges was $73,029, giving total savings in 1978 of $258,285. If, under the more liberal assumption 2, cimetidine is viewed as an intervention that eliminated hospitalization, then total charge savings in Rhode Island in 1978 were $449,846.

These estimates may be extrapolated to the national level by using aggregate U.S. health care expenditures. The total saving at the national level was conservatively estimated as $59,162,500 in 1978 (including $21,150,000 in physician fees) and liberally estimated as $97,175,000. These data projections are given in Table 4.

EPIDEMIOLOGY AND AMBULATORY TREATMENT OF PEPTIC ULCER DISEASE IN RHODE ISLAND

Since hospitalization for ulcer disease is a relatively infrequent event, although admittedly an expensive one, many of the costs of treating ulcer disease have not been adequately investigated. The majority of those with ulcer disease will not be hospitalized, but will incur costs for other medical services, eg, physician visits, diagnostic tests, medications. Other costs to society can also be expected, such as decreased productivity through lost workdays.

A randomly selected population with ulcer disease in Rhode Island was surveyed and an attempt was made to identify all the costs associated with the disease for those who received cimetidine and for those who did not.

Methods

Between February and May, 1980, a health interview survey of 2,258 households in Rhode Island was conducted for the Department of Health. A respondent rate of 93% was obtained (2,097 households and 5,728 individuals). A total of 195

Table 3

Charges for Hospitalization of Rhode Island Blue Cross
and Blue Shield Patients January to June 1976

	Routine charges	Ancillary charges	Blue Shield surgery physicians fees	Total
Partial gastrectomy	$1,775	$1,519	$700	$3,994
Vagotomy	1,824	1,210	535	3,569
Ulcer and ulcer related without ulcer surgery	1,189	465		1,654

Source: Blue Cross and Blue Shield of Rhode Island and CPHA abstracts

Table 4

Rhode Island Hospitalization Cost Savings

		Hospital costs	
	Physician costs	**Reduction* in discharges**	**No reduction* in discharges**
Average cost of ulcer surgery (Rhode Island, 1976 dollars)	$674	$3,252	$1,598
Reduction in surgery per 10,000 population	×0.987	×0.987	×0.987
Population (in 10,000's)	×93.5	×93.5	×93.5
Savings in 1976 dollars	$62,200	$300,109	$147,471
Total expenditure in Rhode Island 1976 (000) (all diseases)	$99,848	$304,235	$304,235
Savings as percent of total expenditure	0.06%	0.10%	0.05%
Rhode Island savings in 1976 dollars	$62,200	$304,154	$147,471
Inflation (1976 to 1978)†	1.177	1.255	1.255
Rhode Island savings in 1978 dollars	$73,209	$376,637	$185,076

United States projection

		Hospital costs	
	Physician costs	**Reduction in discharges**	**No reduction in discharges**
Percent of total expenditure saved in Rhode Island	0.06	0.10	0.05
U.S. expenditures, 1978 (000,000)	$35,250	$76,025	$76,025
U.S. projected savings, 1978 (000,000)	21.150	76.025	38.012

Total U.S. projected savings, 1978

	Liberal estimate	Conservative estimate
Physician costs	$21,150,000	$21,150,000
Hospital costs	76,025,000	38,012,500
Total Savings	$97,175,000	$59,162,500

*Reduction in discharges assumes hospitalization is avoided. No reduction in discharges assumes surgery is avoided but case is treated medically in the hospital.

†CPI physician service index (1976=188.5; 1978=22.18)
 Rhode Island Blue Cross average daily hospital costs (1976=$180.16; 1978=$226.10)

people, 3% of the population, reported an ulcer. Ninety-seven percent of these people granted permission for recontact. This was the ulcer population studied in this survey.

Questionnaires were designed to permit comparisons of health experiences between current cimetidine users and non-users and between pre- and post-cimetidine use. Information was elicited about diagnosis, medication, use of health services, and other variables.

Data collection began June 9, 1980 and ended July 15, 1980. One hundred forty interviews were completed, 52 with cimetidine users and 88 with cimetidine nonusers.

Results

Prevalence of Ulcer Disease. The prevalence of ulcer disease in Rhode Island was estimated in 1975 to be 19.5 per 1,000. In 1980, 25.5 per 1,000 in Rhode Island reported an ulcer. However, when corrections are made for over-reporting, the figure was close to 21 per 1,000, which is not significantly higher than in 1975.

Incidence of Ulcer Disease. The incidence of newly diagnosed ulcers was 2.6 per 1,000, similar to the incidence of 2.9 in 1975 in the National Health Survey.

Medication Regimen. Forty-one percent reported using cimetidine, and 59% reported that they had never used the drug. Three general types of nonusers were identified: 1) those with unconfirmed ulcer who were self-medicated, 2) those with a confirmed ulcer who were self-medicated, and 3) those with confirmed ulcer who had recently been under a physician's care. This last category was the appropriate comparison group in this study, since cimetidine users are under a physician's care. The final numbers for the study were 44 users and 31 never-users of cimetidine, all 75 had physician-confirmed duodenal or unspecified peptic ulcer and had seen a physician in the past 2 years.

Characteristics of Users and Nonusers. The two groups are quite different. Users tended to be female, over 45 years, and have family incomes over $15,000. They were more likely to be working full- or part-time and less likely to be homemakers, retired, or students. Users were generally healthier also, although not necessarily with less than severe ulcers. They were less likely than nonusers to report depressions, limited activity, or other chronic conditions. Both groups had the same number of physician visits per year, although non-users had more difficulty obtaining medical care than their user counterparts.

Users were more likely than nonusers to have had their ulcers confirmed.

Respondents reported varying use of cimetidine: from one to four tablets per day during 1 week to 1 year. Users' compliance with prescriptions was significantly higher than nonusers'. Both groups saw physicians with approximately the same regularity. The hospitalization rate for ulcer disease, higher for the user group, was based on one patient and must be interpreted with caution.

Users reported significantly fewer bed days at home (1.1) and disability days (4.5) for ulcer disease than nonusers (1.8 and 11.3, respectively).

Changes in Health Status. Since the user and nonuser groups are very different, a comparison of their ulcer experience would suffer because drug use would be only one of the many variables possibly explaining differences between the two groups. There is considerable evidence, however, that the health of users improved after cimetidine intervention while nonusers showed less improvement. Of the users, 83% reported an improved ulcer condition; 17% reported no change; none reported deterioration. Of nonusers, 30% reported the ulcer was worse; 37% reported it was better; 33% reported no change. Along with the greater improvement in the cimetidine groups were corresponding reductions in the utilization of health services. These are shown in Tables 5 and 6.

Cost Implications. Users were found to incur lower costs overall than nonusers, as shown in Table 7. The cost of disability days for users was much lower. Costs of disease prior to cimetidine were not assignable, but it is clear that a reduction occurred. Cimetidine users almost uniformly reported an improvement in their disease, and the majority reported a decrease in utilization of services after cimetidine intervention. Nonusers, on the other hand, were just as likely to have increased as decreased utilization (and presumably costs) during the past 2 years.

Summary

User and nonuser groups were quite different in general health and in utilization patterns. However, there is a marked improvement in ulcer disease and

---

Table 5

Changes in Utilization of Health Services After Cimetidine Intervention (Group A)

Use of other medications (N = 34)	
Use more after cimetidine	3%
Use less after cimetidine	79%
Use the same	17%
	100%*
Physician visits (N = 28)	
More after cimetidine	0%
Fewer after cimetidine	57%
Same	43%
	100%
Telephone calls to physicians (N = 17)	
More after cimetidine	0%
Fewer after cimetidine	82%
Same	18%
	100%
Hospitalization rate per 100 years ulcer experience	
Before cimetidine	6.3 (N = 317 years)
After cimetidine	1.4 (N = 69.3 years)

*Totals may not equal 100% due to rounding

a marked decrease in utilization of services following cimetidine therapy. Cimetidine non-users were less likely than users to report an improvement in health status or a decrease in utilization.

Table 6

Changes in Utilization of Health Services During the Past 2 Years (Group B)

Comparing use of medication
last year and 2 years ago (N = 29)

Use more now	34%
Use less now	45%
Same	21%
	100%

Physician visits (N = 29)

More now	40%
Fewer now	37%
Same	23%
	100%

Telephone calls to physicians
(N = 8)

More now	25%
Fewer now	75%
Same	0%
	100%

Hospitalization rate per 100 years
ulcer experience   2.2 (N = 312 years)

WORK LOSS DUE TO ULCER DISEASE IN RHODE ISLAND

All private employees and some self-employed individuals in Rhode Island are covered by Temporary Disability Insurance (TDI). Payments are made to individuals missing 7 or more consecutive days of work because of illness. Duodenal and gastric ulcer are not differentiated.

Ulcer claims per 1,000 covered employees and as a percent of all claims were not significantly different in 1978 than in 1977. The data are in Table 8. Results of this aspect of the survey lead the authors to conclude that there was not a significant acceleration of the trend in declining work-loss rates for peptic ulcer disease as might have been expected after the introduction of cimetidine.

Table 7

Costs Associated with Ulcer Disease for Group A and Group B

	Average annual cost	
	Group A	**Group B**
Cimetidine	$79	$0
Other medications	45	54
Physician visits	47	30
Bed and disability days	139	325
	$310	$409

Table 8

Work-Loss Claims due to Peptic Ulcer Disease Reported by the Rhode Island Temporary Disability Insurance Program*

Year	Covered employees	Total claims	Peptic ulcer claims	Ulcer claims per 1,000 covered employees	Ulcer as percent of all claims
1974	307,022	43,779	610	1.987	1.4%
1975	289,900	38,639	503	1.735	1.3
1976	307,678	40,140	453	1.472	1.1
1977	322,219	39,870	421	1.307	1.1
1978	339,257	40,519	375	1.105	0.9
1979	345,035	43,285	395	1.145	0.9

*The claims are for workers who have been unable to work for 7 consecutive days
Source: Rhode Island Temporary Disability Insurance Program

10.

Bulthuis R:

Surgery trends and the costs of peptic ulcer disease before and after the introduction of cimetidine.

Economisch Statistische Berichten 25:292–293, 1981; and *Cimetidine, Surgery Trends and the Cost of Peptic Ulcer Disease*, Symposium, Amsterdam, March 20, 1981 (proceedings in press)

In 1979, the cost of health care in the Netherlands was 26 billion guilders, 8.6% of GNP. Factors other than government policies can help to reduce health care costs; cimetidine, an example of technological progress, is one such factor.

THE CHANGING COST OF PEPTIC ULCER DISEASE

The cost of peptic ulcer disease to the Dutch economy rose, in current prices, from 49 million to 88.5 million guilders in the years from 1972 to 1979. This 80% increase is significantly smaller than the 120% rise in total health care costs in the same period and the 170% rise in the cost of the average hospital day. What is the reason for this "lag" or relative decline in total ulcer costs?

EVOLUTION OF PEPTIC ULCER DISEASE COSTS

The costs of peptic ulcer can be separated into three categories: hospital costs including surgery, out-patient costs including consultations and diagnostic procedures, and medicine costs.

MEDICINE COSTS

Medicine costs for peptic ulcer disease have shown a dramatic rise, increasing sixfold between 1972 and 1979, with the steepest rise beginning in 1977 coincident with the introduction of cimetidine.

OUTPATIENT COSTS

The decisive factor in the 130% increase in out-patient costs for peptic ulcer disease is technological change, namely the advent of the fiber-optic endoscope. This cost increase took place gradually in the years after 1974.

HOSPITAL COSTS

The relative decline in total ulcer disease costs took place in hospital costs. Hospital costs for peptic ulcer rose "only" 54% from 1972 to 1979. The number of hospital days for peptic ulcer disease declined by 40% (153,000 days), while the cost per hospital day for ulcer patients rose 170%. The decline in hospital days fully accounts for the decline in hospital costs. Two thirds of this cost change is due to a reduction in number of admissions and one third to a reduction in average length of stay.

ULCER SURGERY

The number of hospital admissions for duodenal ulcer who did not undergo surgery declined by 38 percent from 4,700 to 2,900 in the period 1972 to 1979. A sharp decline in such admissions from 4,500 in 1974 to 3,800 in 1975 and a second from 3,700 in 1977 to 3,300 in 1978 are noteworthy. The number of patients admitted for gastric ulcer who did not undergo surgery also declined over the same period but not as dramatically. In contrast to the decline in the number of hospital admissions for gastric and duodenal ulcer patients who did not undergo surgery, the number of all admissions to hospitals in the Netherlands has risen steadily since 1972.

Patients admitted to hospital for peptic ulcer (gastric and duodenal ulcer) who underwent surgery in the period 1972 to 1979 followed quite a different pattern. The number of partial gastrectomies and vagotomies for duodenal ulcer performed annually remained quite stable at around 3,000 between 1972 and 1977, but after the introduction of cimetidine dropped suddenly to 2,300 in 1978 and declined further to 2,100 in 1979. The annual number of partial gastrectomies and vagotomies performed for gastric ulcer also dropped suddenly from 1,700 in 1977 to 1,200 in 1978 after a slight decline in the period to 1977. See Figures 1 and 2.

ANALYSIS OF CAUSE USING REGRESSION ANALYSIS

The trend in the annual number of admissions for peptic ulcer disease who underwent surgery is in complete contrast with the steady annual increase

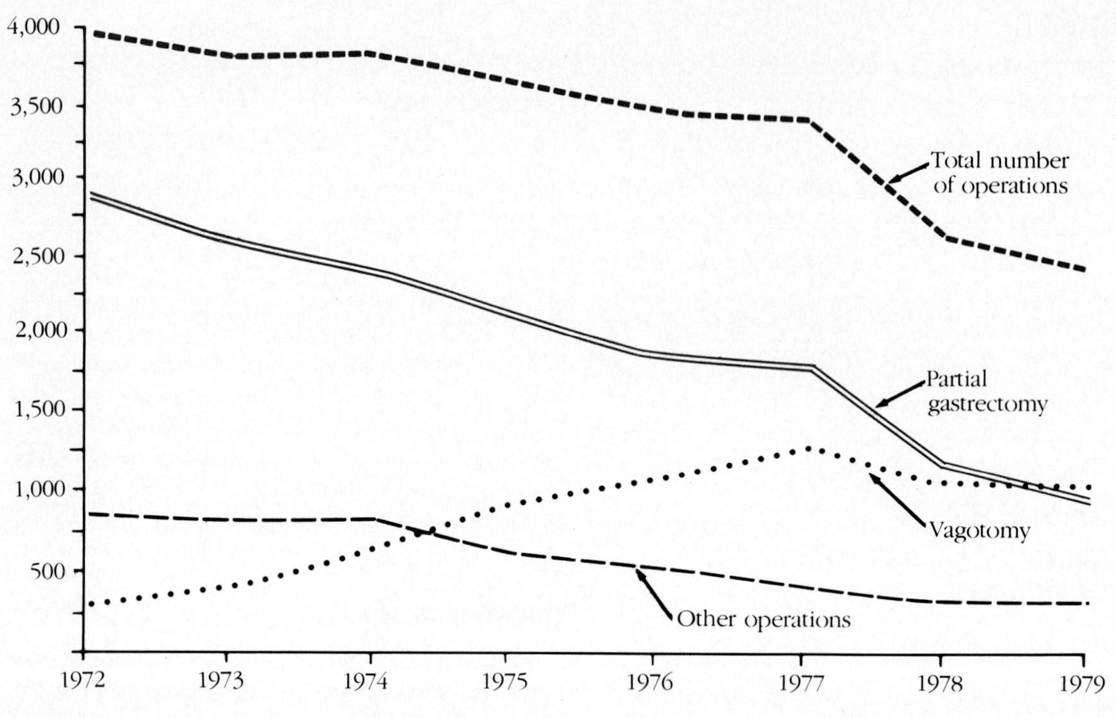

Figure 1. Trend in the number of *operated* hospitalizations for *duodenal ulcer* by type of operation.

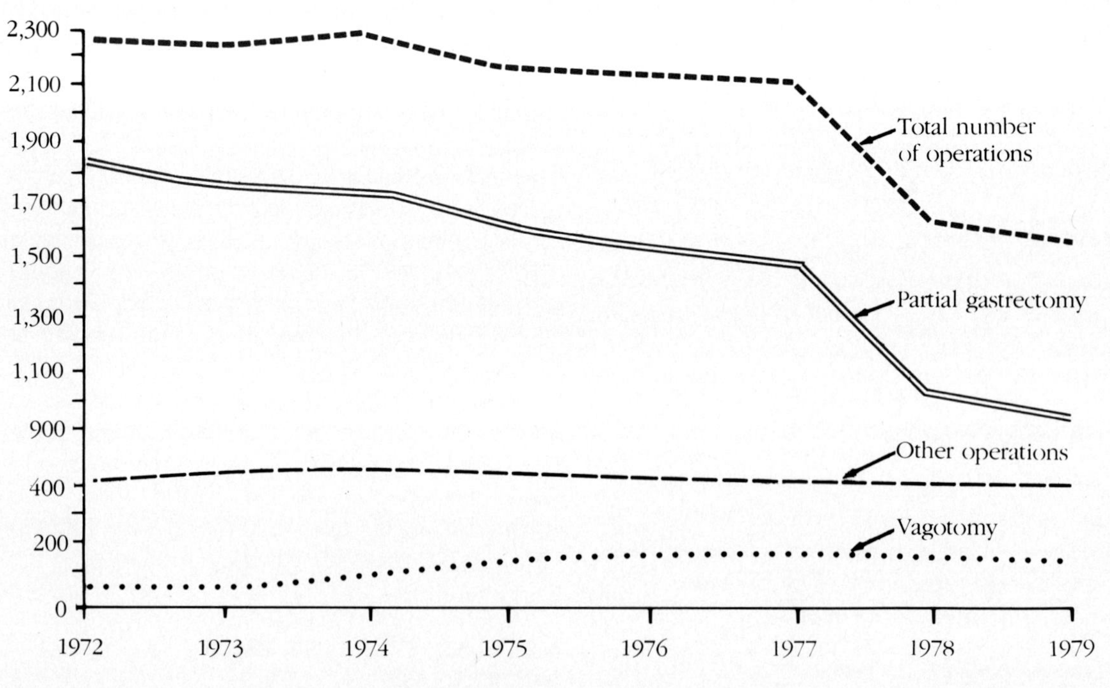

Figure 2. Trend in the number of *operated* hospitalizations for *gastric ulcer* by type of operation.

Table

The Reduction in the Number of Hospital Admissions for Peptic Ulcer Disease Attributable
to the Established Trend and to Cimetidine

	Gastric ulcer		Duodenal ulcer		Peptic ulcer (total)	
	Cimetidine	Trend	Cimetidine	Trend	Cimetidine	Trend
Hospital admissions without surgery	n.a.	300	n.a.	1,700	n.a.	2,000
Hospital admissions with partial gastrectomy or vagotomy	400	400	1,000	n.a.	1,400	400
Hospital admissions with 'other' operations	n.a.	n.a.	n.a.	500	n.a.	500
Total	400	700	1,000	2,200	1,400	2,900

n.a. = no admission

in the number of all admissions to Netherland hospitals who underwent surgery in the period 1972 to 1979. Examination of the possible causal factors by regression analysis shows that only two factors, the drug cimetidine and the "annual trend" achieve statistical significance. Of the 1,800 fewer admissions for peptic ulcer disease who underwent surgery, 1,400 of the decline are attributable to cimetidine and 400 to "trend." On the other hand, the 2,000 decline in admissions for patients who did not undergo surgery is attributable to "trend," with cimetidine not achieving statistical causal significance (Table).

MONEY COSTS

Translated into monetary terms, of the 43.5-million-guilder "lag" in peptic ulcer hospital costs relative to the increase in total (surgical and non-surgical) hospital costs, 33.5 million is attributable to established trend and 10 million to cimetidine.

When the 5.5-million-guilder increase in medicine costs due to cimetidine expenditures is considered, the net effect of cimetidine is a 4.5 million guilder saving.

CONCLUSION

From 1972 to 1979, the fundamental cost structure for peptic ulcer disease has changed in the Netherlands. On a relative basis, medicine and out-patient costs have increased, largely due to the expenditures on cimetidine and endoscopy. Total ulcer costs have, in contrast, relatively declined because of a greater reduction in hospital costs induced by the effects of cimetidine and to some extent of "annual trend."

It may be stated, then, that efficacious new medications can actually save treatment costs for the nation. The availability of the computerized data and the isolation techniques of regression analysis make these conclusions possible.

11.

Geweke JF, Weisbrod BA:
Some economic consequences of technological advance in medical care: The case of a new drug, in Helms RB (ed): Drugs and Health. Economic Issues and Policy Objectives.
Washington and London, American Enterprise Institute for Public Policy Research, 1981, pp 235–271

In a study published in the recent book *Drugs and Health*,* two health economists at the University of Wisconsin draw the following conclusion from their analysis of some 1,200 patients' records in Texas Medicaid's computer files:

> From the narrow viewpoint of minimizing government expenditure the question is, which alternative or combination involves the lowest level of expenditure. We have not compared all possible treatment combinations, but what we have found is that using cimetidine does appear to reduce expenditures on treatment of duodenal ulcers compared to the average of other treatment technologies not employing cimetidine.

The authors found that an average duodenal ulcer episode treated with cimetidine cost Medicaid 11 to 63% less in reimbursement payments than did an episode not treated with cimetidine. The exact percentage depends on what cost items and treatment periods are considered; however, all combinations are positive for cimetidine.

The savings from cimetidine for the different cost items and treatment periods in the study are summarized in Table 1. The reader must question what the savings would be if drugs and all other cost components (nursing homes, etc), not just the larger inpatient and physician costs, were included in the ulcer-specific view. If these missing components are assumed on a worst-case basis, the 63 and 40% become respectively 48 and 23% savings in total ulcer-specific costs. (These worst-case savings, derived from the study, are not specifically cited by the authors.)

METHODOLOGY

Inferences about socioeconomic effects must be drawn in nonexperimental settings, often by using data bases that have not been constructed for such purposes. The authors believe that the methodology used here was general enough to be used for any drug, although the focus was on the use of cimetidine in duodenal ulcers. All the data used in this study were taken from Medicaid claims in the state of Texas for the period September, 1976 through June, 1978. The most attractive feature of this data base relative to others is the availability of detailed medical information about the period in which health care costs were incurred as well as the

---

Table 1

Range of Percent Savings From Cimetidine for the Average Duodenal Ulcer Patient (Under Age 65)

All conditions view (considers all conditions, not just ulcer, and all costs)	Ulcer-specific, key-costs view (considers only treatment specifically for ulcer and only inpatients and physician costs)
First-month view	
During the first (+1) month after drug prescribed for the ulcer 25%	63%
Three-month view	
During the first month prior (−1) through second month after (+2) drug prescribed for the ulcer 11%	40%

---

*Helms RB (ed): *Drugs and Health. Economic Issues and Policy Objectives.* Washington and London, American Enterprise Institute for Public Policy Research, 1981.

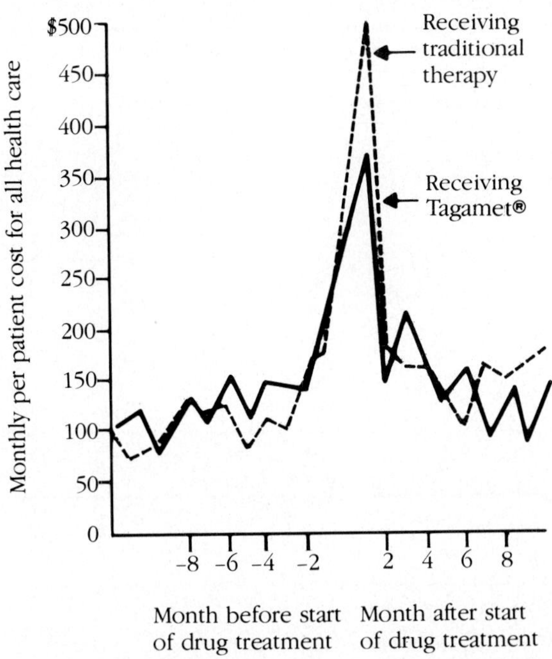

Figure. The cost to Medicaid of an average duodenal ulcer patient (under age 65). Interpretation: During the first month after drug treatment started, duodenal ulcer patients treated with cimetidine incurred average expenditures for all health care that were 25% lower per patient than those of similar patients on other forms of therapy ($506 – $381 = $125 ÷ $506 = 25%).

time at which they were billed. Together with the availability of patient identification numbers, this information makes possible a detailed reconstruction of that portion of a patient's health care history paid for by the state. Unfortunately, this means that only direct costs billable to the Medicaid system were known and there was no information on severity or mortality.

The basic comparisons in this study are between duodenal ulcer patients who received cimetidine at some time between September 1, 1977, and June 30, 1978 and all other duodenal ulcer patients who received treatment but not cimetidine at some time during the same period.

RESULTS: FIRST-MONTH VIEWS

One meaningful view considers all health care costs (including those for concomitant conditions, not just for the ulcer) during the first-month after the start of drug therapy. This view, finding first month savings of 25%, appears in simplified form in the Figure.

Introductory sections of the study explain how the cimetidine and non-cimetidine patients were grouped on the basis of similar pretreatment costs so that disease severity and other factors were equalized as far as possible. This controls for a patient selection bias in the data: toward cimetidine for the more severe patients.

The overall savings graphed in the Figure come mainly from lower hospital inpatient and physician costs, as shown by the data in Table 2 (provided

Table 2

First-Month All-Conditions Cost to Medicaid for an Average Duodenal Ulcer Patient (Under Age 65)

	378 patients receiving cimetidine	**482 patients receiving other therapy**	**Savings with cimetidine**
Cost components			
Hospital inpatient	$219	$347	$128 (37%)
Physician	94	106	12 (1%)
Drugs	32	15*	-17 (-111%)
Hospital outpatient	18	15	-3 (-20%)
Nursing home	11	13	2 (15%)
Other	8	10	2
Total cost	$381	$506	$125 (25%)

*Traditional drug treatment for ulcer typically employs antacids in daily doses too low to heal the ulcer as efficiently as cimetidine does. If antacid doses therapeutically equivalent to cimetidine were used (for example, 14 oz of Maalox® Suspension per day) the cost at the time of the study would have exceeded $1.85 per day. Cimetidine at that time cost $1.30 per day. Significant at the 5% level or less: $128, -$17, and $125; other differences not significant at the 10% level. (For the readers who have forgotten their statistics, significance at the 5% level means that the difference between the two groups would be found by chance only 5 times in 100; the 1% level means it would be found by chance only 1 time in 100.)

Table 3

First-Month Ulcer-Specific Costs to Medicaid for an Average Duodenal Ulcer Patient (Under Age 65)

Cost components	378 patients receiving cimetidine	482 patients receiving other therapy	Savings with cimetidine
Hospital inpatient Physician	$102	$279	$177 (63%)*
Drugs Hospital outpatient Nursing home Other	} †		
Total cost†			

*The $177 is significant at the 1% level.
†Information not available.

Table 4

Worst Case: First-Month Ulcer-Specific Costs to Medicaid for an
Average Duodenal Ulcer Patient (Under Age 65)

	Cost components	378 patients receiving cimetidine	482 patients receiving other therapy	Savings with cimetidine
	Hospital inpatient Physician	$102	$279	$177
Worst case	Drugs	32	15	–17
	Hospital inpatient	18	15	–3
	Nursing home	11	13	2
	Other	8	10	2
	Total cost	$171	$332	$161 (48%)

supplementally by the authors). Hospital inpatient costs were reduced by $128, more than enough to offset the cost increases. Note that drug costs increased with cimetidine by $17. The net outcome was the $125 or 25% saving graphed in the Figure.

Another more restricted but possibly more relevant view of the first month data considers only the hospital inpatient and physician cost components and, within these components, only costs identified as due specifically to the ulcer itself and not to other conditions. Since other conditions often appear with ulcer, especially among the severe or costly patients, this restricted view is appropriate, even though potentially costly items such as drugs are not included. This can be allowed for as shown in Table 3, which indicates a savings of 63% for the cimetidine group.

Unfortunately, ulcer-specific costs are sufficiently identified in the patient records only for hospital inpatient care and physician services; and the two categories are lumped in the study. Fortunately, these are the two most important cost components, being the largest in Table 2, and thus provide a strong indication of the total ulcer-specific cost outcome. For example, it is clear that the $177 inpatient-plus-physician saving from cimetidine is more than enough to offset the $17 increase in drug costs for *all* conditions noted in Table 2.

In fact, to test a worst-case result one might fill in the ulcer-specific costs missing in Table 3 with the all-conditions costs from Table 2—knowing that the ulcer-specific costs are contained within the all-conditions costs. (In other words, we assume the ulcer is responsible for all treatment the patient receives.) The result is still positive for cimetidine (Table 4).

We see that the average duodenal ulcer episode treated with cimetidine cost Medicaid at least 48% less in payments for first-month ulcer-specific treatment than did an episode not treated with cimetidine.

RESULTS: THREE-MONTH VIEWS

Geweke and Weisbrod write that the first-month view just presented (excluding the worst-case view, which they do not consider) understates the treatment costs caused by cimetidine and thus may overstate the savings it produces. This is because some medical measures, such as endoscopy to confirm a diagnosis of duodenal ulcer, were probably taken in the month prior to the cimetidine prescription as precautions before using the new technology. Thus, costs in month –1 as well as +1 should be counted in the ulcer episode. Likewise, costs in the second month (+2) may well reflect the treatment effects of cimetidine and should also be counted. Thus, a three-month period (–1 through +2) is an appropriate alternative view. However, it is an alternative and not necessarily a better view, the authors feel, since including month –1 probably overstates the cimetidine-related costs relative to those of non-cimetidine treatment.

The 3-month views (Tables 5 and 6) show an 11 and a 40% cost saving with cimetidine, and a 23% saving under the worst-case ulcer-specific assumption. Again, the $114 saving is more than enough to offset cost increases, as seen when the all-conditions cost increases from Table 5 are

Table 5

Three-Month All-Conditions Costs to Medicaid for an Average Duodenal Ulcer Patient (Under Age 65)

Cost components	356 patients receiving cimetidine	449 patients receiving other therapy	Savings with cimetidine
Hospital inpatient	$433	$521	$88 (17%)
Physician	169	193	24 (12%)
Drugs	61	35	–26 (–74%)*
Hospital outpatient	39	30	–9 (–30%)
Nursing home	33	43	10 (23%)
Other	17	24	7 (29%)
Total cost	$752	$846	$94 (23%)

*Significant at the 1% level:–$26; other differences not significant at the 10% level.

Table 6

Three-Month Ulcer-Specific Costs to Medicaid for an Average Duodenal Ulcer Patient (Under Age 65)

Cost components	356 patients receiving cimetidine	449 patients receiving other therapy	Savings with cimetidine
Hospital inpatient Physician	$172	$286	$114 (40%)*
Drugs Hospital outpatient Nursing home Other	} †		
Total cost†			

* The $114 is significant at the 5% level.
† Information not available.

Worst Case: Three-Month Ulcer-Specific Costs to Medicaid for an
Average Duodenal Ulcer Patient (Under Age 65)

		356 patients receiving cimetidine	449 patients receiving other therapy	Savings with cimetidine
	Cost components			
	Hospital inpatient Physician	$172	$286	$114
Worst case	Drugs	61	35	–26
	Hospital inpatient	39	30	–9
	Nursing home	33	43	10
	Other	17	24	7
	Total cost	$322	$418	$96 (23%)

inserted in a worst-case example—ie, assuming all treatment costs the patient generates are due specifically to the ulcer (Table 7).

Thus, the average duodenal ulcer episode treated with cimetidine cost Medicaid at least 23% less in reimbursement payments for three-month ulcer-specific treatment than did an episode not treated with cimetidine.

12.

Culyer AJ, Maynard AK:
Cost-effectiveness of duodenal ulcer treatment.
Social Science and Medicine 15c:3–11, 1981

Experience at several English hospitals suggests that one third of ulcer patients who would formerly have been operated on have indications of long-term cimetidine use as the preferred method of clinical management. In clinical trials cimetidine has always produced greater healing than placebo. However, clinical and cost-effectiveness comparisons with surgery have not been done and seem to be a gap in our knowledge.

LIMITATIONS OF PREVIOUS TRIALS

The existing literature on cimetidine trials is found lacking for several reasons: (1) testing cimetidine in non-controlled or open trials casts doubt on the results versus alternative treatment; (2) testing in placebo-controlled trials can establish dose, optimal duration of treatment, and superiority of cimetidine to placebo, but the benefit and cost relative to other realistic treatments are not

established; and (3) though surgery is the only method that will reverse the ulcer problem in most patients, long-term comparison of results versus cimetidine have not been studied clinically.

EVALUATION OF COSTS

As leading contenders for treatment choice, surgery and cimetidine merit economic evaluation as well. Economic evaluation is concerned with the decisional question "is something worthwhile doing," a question which invites many further questions, of which two are "worthwhile relative to what alternative?" and "worthwhile to whom?" Ideally, a complete economic evaluation should take account of the benefits as well as the costs—ie, the changed state of health or well-being of the patient. However, because this is difficult to measure and express in money terms, the kind of economic evaluation in this study is cost-effectiveness analysis. Preferably, a cost-effectiveness analysis should compare only alternatives that lead to similar outcomes. Thus, a working assumption of the present study is that cimetidine and surgery are equally satisfactory in health outcomes. Typically outcomes are not identical; some symptomatic relief is more complete than others, or some treatments may take effect sooner. Thus the "least cost" method may not be the best choice if higher cost methods produce superior outcomes.

TRUE SOCIAL COSTS

The total social costs of a treatment must be evaluated in the broadest context without sectorial boundaries. Private, public, and family interest should be included. Also, focus should shift from *expenditure flows* to *real cost flows*. Potentially this is the most revolutionary concept, since it may involve attributing costs in the nonmarketed sector such as the value of family members' time. It also involves the critical appraisal of market prices and other factors such as transfer payments.

SURGICAL TREATMENT

The surgical costs of duodenal ulcer are institutional costs to hospitals, time costs to patients, and costs associated with death from surgery.

HOSPITAL COSTS

These costs can be calculated by taking the average length of hospital stay for vagotomy patients and multiplying it by the average cost per day, by deriving marginal costs of surgery cases with a regression model of hospital costs, or by estimating the costs directly in a representative major treatment center. The results for the Newcastle Royal Victoria Infirmary are displayed in Table 1 and have been used in this analysis. (These costs represent averages, found to be close to marginal cost figures and confirming 400 as the approximate true cost of a vagotomy to the hospital in 1978.)

PATIENT COSTS

Patient costs are not a part of any public budget but may be substantial and must be counted when evaluated from the point of view of the community. In this study, patient costs are limited to loss of earnings attributable to surgery versus cimetidine treatment. Using the results of an American study, the authors estimate that the return to work is from

Table 1

Hospital Costs of Vagotomy as Estimated in Newcastle Royal Victoria Infirmary 1978 (£)

Ward costs per patient-day	Lowest estimate	Highest estimate
Medical staff time	4.66	5.08
Nursing staff time	9.71	10.26
Other	6.69	6.69
Total	21.06	22.03
Total ward costs per case (row 4 × 16.1)	339.07	354.68
Operating costs per case	33.65	45.25
Total hospital costs per case (row 5 + row 6)	372.72	399.93

Notes

1. 16.1 days is the national average length of stay for vagotomy; in Newcastle the range was from 10 to 21 days.

2. Medical staff costs: a House Officer was on duty at all times and this doctor was supervised by a Registrar. While the House Officer was on duty at all times in unit he was able to perform tasks. The hourly cost of the doctor was calculated taking the median salary dividing it by 52 and 40 (52 weeks, 40 hours per week), and then multiplying it by 24 (ie it was assumed that the House Officer spent 24 of his 40 weekly working hours working in the unit). We assumed that senior staff spent one half of their time working in the unit. Alternative assumptions about sick leave and holidays were made and gave rise to the high and low estimates in Table 2.

3. Nursing costs: various combinations of nursing staff were employed in the unit eg, two SRNs, one SEN and five student nurses, or two SENs, one SRN and five students (two or three of whom might be in their third year of training). The staffing information was combined with the Treasurer's estimates of the costs of 1 hour of nursing time. This cost is made up of the basic salary, enhancements, national health insurance and super-annuation. Median values were used for all grades. Alternative assumptions about sickness leave (2 or 4 weeks) and holidays (including and excluding them) were made to generate alternative hourly cost estimates. Length of stay data were provided by the consultant.

4. Other costs: fire, light, power, water, cleaning. Porterage and food costs were estimated from data provided by the Treasurer.

5. Operating costs: staffing was assumed to consist of two SRNs, one student nurse, two house officers, one consultant surgeon, and one consultant anesthetist. It was assumed that one house officer was paid at the bottom rate of the house officer scale and one senior house officer (SHO) was paid at the bottom rate of the SHO scale. It was assumed that both consultants were paid at the lowest consultant grade rate.

30 to 50% faster with cimetidine than with surgery. In 1978 these assumptions—weighted for male and female earnings (including housewives' opportunity wage)—yield time costs of £584 and £974, respectively. These are minimal, for they do not include the cost of pain, nor the hidden costs falling on family members, nor the costs falling on primary-care and local-authority services.

CASE FATALITY COSTS

Since cimetidine reduces the probability of surgery, which carries a small but positive probability of death, one benefit of cimetidine lies in its effect on case fatalities. The kinds of ulcer surgery in the U.K. likely to be replaced by cimetidine are the lesser uncomplicated procedures, vagotomies with or without pyloroplasty, for which one study reported a 0.5% fatality rate. This is low according to some authorities. The authors use this low figure, again possibly understating the costs of surgery.

Though an emotional issue, the value of a human life can be calculated in three ways. The social decisions method infers from public actions about lifesaving expenditure what was the minimum value on preventing a single statistical death. This value varies greatly; the Department of the Environment put it at £68,500. The human capital method discounts the value of all future earnings (gross of income tax) and, at 7% for 25 years, yields £46,000. Nonearners are ignored. The risk avoidance method establishes the maximum amount an individual would pay to effect a set reduction in the probability of death. The most rigorous study of this last type derived a mean value of £3 million—larger by far than the other estimates and, perhaps, more in accord with intuition.

Using these alternative estimates and the minimum case fatality rate of 0.5%, the implied costs per surgery are £230, £340, and £15,000 in ascending order. Table 2 then summarizes the total cost per surgical patient.

CIMETIDINE TREATMENT

The costs of cimetidine are relatively straightforward. Case fatality is absent. Adverse effects are assumed absent: an assumption that seems to the authors in accord with experience to date but which may need modification after experience with long-term maintenance. The costs of medical supervision by general practitioners have been assumed trivial enough to be ignored. Diagnostic procedures that are common to both medical and surgical treatment are omitted. The two cost patterns for cimetidine (Table 3) were developed for discount rates (needed to give present values of expenditures in the future) of 5%, 7%, and 10%. Pattern 1 consisted of 1 gram per day for 4 weeks, followed by a maintenance on 400 milligrams per day. Pattern 2 consisted of 1 gram per day for 6 weeks and 400 milligrams per day thereafter. Each treatment pattern was examined for ages 20, 25, 30, and 35 years.

Table 2

Costs per Case of Surgical Treatment of Duodenal Ulcer by Vagotomy (1978 Prices)

	Lowest estimate	Highest estimate
Ward costs	340	350
Operating costs	30	50
Differential patient costs	580	970
Value of risk of death	230	15,000
Total cost per case	1,180	16,370

Table 3

Cost of Two Patterns of Long-Term Cimetidine Treatment (£ per Case)

| | Duration of treatment | | | | | | | | | | | |
	20 years			25 years			30 years			35 years		
Discount rate (%)	5	7	10	5	7	10	5	7	10	5	7	10
Pattern 1												
Present value of first year's cost	100	98	96	100	98	96	100	98	96	100	98	96
Present value of subsequent year's cost	1,085	911	717	1,239	1,011	770	1,360	1,082	807	1,454	1,132	823
Total	1,185	1,009	813	1,339	1,109	866	1,460	1,180	903	1,554	1,230	919
Pattern 2												
Present value of first year's cost	109	107	104	109	107	104	109	107	104	109	107	104
Present value of subsequent year's cost	1,085	911	717	1,239	1,011	770	1,360	1,082	807	1,454	1,132	823
Total	1,194	1,018	821	1,348	1,118	874	1,469	1,189	911	1,563	1,239	927

A price of 12.95 pence per 200 mg of cimetidine is used

Treatment pattern 1 consists of 1,000 mg per day for 4 weeks and 400 mg per day thereafter

Treatment pattern 2 consists of 1,000 mg per day for 6 weeks and 400 mg per day thereafter

Table 4

Summary of Cost per Case of Vagotomy and
Cimetidine

	Lowest estimate	Highest estimate
Vagotomy	1,180	16,370
Cimetidine	1,010	1,240

RESULTS

The range of cost estimates just overlaps (Table 4), with the highest estimate of drug costs just exceeding the lowest of the vagotomy estimates. However, cost estimates have overstated the likely cost of drug therapy for an average patient and have systematically understated the cost of surgery. Bearing this in mind, the authors judge drug treatment to be substantially less costly than vagotomy for duodenal ulcer.

This conclusion assumes the public sector discount rate of 7%. The choice of rate affects the relative costliness of the two procedures, the lower the rate chosen the greater the relative costliness of cimetidine. Noting, however, the desirability of using a consistent discount rate in public sector decisions and noting the inadequate basis for risking deaths from operation—a basis which seriously understates these costs in the authors' opinion—the study again concludes with the judgment that drug treatment with cimetidine is substantially less costly than surgery for duodenal ulcer where the choice is clinically acceptable.

DISCUSSION

This study is not a *cost-benefit* study but rather a *cost-effectiveness* study that is valid only if the outcomes are sufficiently close in terms of human welfare. Also, the alternatives considered are a fraction of the total alternative treatments available. The prices in the analysis have been accepted fairly uncritically, and the impact of *unknown* costs cannot be told. The adverse effects of years of cimetidine therapy have yet to be described and quantitated.

From Table 2, it can be calculated that patient costs contribute 49% of the lowest surgical costs and the value-of-life cost contributes 92% of the highest surgical cost estimate. With neither of these costs considered, the highest surgical cost is only about £400 per case—about half the cost of the drugs in the cimetidine regimen. From the NHS point of view, surgery seems the cheaper alternative, whereas from the community perspective, surgery is relatively expensive.

APPENDIX D

Policy Interviews

Federal Policy Interviews— Medical Technology Decision Making: A Telephone Survey

David Banta, M.D.

Assistant Director
Office of Technology Assessment
U.S. Congress
Washington, D.C.

Question: What type of policy decisions are made by your department?

Dr. Banta: We really do not make any policy decisions. We are a research and analytical arm of the Congress. We have no decision-making authority except how to spend our own money and even that is somewhat limited. We do make decisions on which studies to undertake concerning medical technology.

Question: How is policy concerning medical technology set?

Dr. Banta: In regards to which study we should undertake, we are continually talking to people both within our agency and outside, such as the staff from the congressional and executive branches. We always have a more or less formal list of possible projects to undertake. This list is checked as we come to the end of a project and then double-checked against what the congressional staff feels are priorities as they would define them. For the most part, they think our ideas are pretty reasonable, but occasionally a new subject will come up. If the person bringing up the subject is important and it seems to be something we can undertake, then we'll usually follow what the person wants. But for the most part, we're very much involved in selecting what we will do.

Question: What steps must occur before a decision is made?

Dr. Banta: Once this informal process has finished, the formal process starts. The chairman of the particular congressional committee that wants the study writes a formal letter that describes the study, sends it to our Congressional Board or to the Director, and then we're formally asked if we have

the money and if we can do it. We then prepare a grant-type proposal that the Congressional Board approves.

Question: What barriers, constraints, problems are faced in trying to establish new policies concerning medical technology?

Dr. Banta: First and foremost, politics. We have a particular system of delivering health care and evaluating technology and there's tremendous inertia built into that system. The system was constructed that way for good reasons, but making any change at all is difficult, and it is a high-risk situation for a group to push for a major change. An enormous number of actors have a large stake in what the system does, and they resist having much done with it.

Information is lacking on the value of specific technologies, on the risk/benefit of specific technologies, and the risk/benefit in relation to cost. Also, there are limitations on what we know about the functioning of the programs that are in place. It's difficult to propose a change in existing policies because we don't know what the effect of the past policies has been.

Question: Who is involved in the total process?

Dr. Banta: Each program, such as basic research, evaluative studies, clinical trials, adoption and use of technology and so on, is subject to its own political pressures and has its own interest groups. Some of the pressure comes from upstairs, that is, the White House and even Congress. It's a complex, dynamic process.

Health care researchers have been basically invisible throughout. I'm personally disappointed in how little the people doing health care research have tried to propose changes in existing policies. The biomedical researchers have been much more successful than the health care providers, who largely function through their interest groups. Traditionally, the most important researchers have been the AMA and the AAMC, representing the academic providers, and the American Hospital Association for the institutional providers, but now we're seeing a tremendous fragmentation. There are so many different groups with which we must deal that it is a pretty confusing situation. Also, manufacturers have become more active in the last few years.

Question: Where do you fit into the process? What role do you play?

Dr. Banta: I hope that we are a little island of objectivity and rationality. Within a highly political environment, we are pretty well insulated from politics, and we really strive to give Congress the facts and options that fall within some bounds of political possibility. We also provide analysis and alternatives to the Congress regarding what it could consider and what the possibilities are. We really have no tie to any program or power, which makes us, I think, unique in the Federal Government. This gives us the possibility of being objective.

Question: How are costs, risks, and benefits of a medical technology evaluated in the process?

Dr. Banta: Well, that is complicated from our point of view. Drugs are examined in a rather systematic fashion through the FDA process of staged clinical trials. Risk and benefit are assessed, but there is no place for cost. A similar program was started in 1976 for medical devices and is more technical than for drugs. Risks are evaluated and determinations are made on whether a device works and does what it's supposed to do.

Nor is there much evaluation of clinical benefits of procedures in this program. There's no systematic approach for procedures.

Question: How might research results be used to aid decision makers?

Dr. Banta: Since research results should be looked at as powerful and useful information, decision makers should become more involved in obtaining that information. I think the key decision makers in this society are the practicing physicians, and these people are not receiving the information they need to make their decisions.

The most change has occurred in the reimbursement programs, particularly Medicare, where the information from evaluations is being used more and more as the basis for coverage decisions. These programs will also be the ones to change the most in the next 5 years.

Our agency is asked to look at the implications of medical technology and over and over again what I find is that the scientific data are inadequate to draw a conclusion. So Congress says, "Should we pay for this or not?" And my answer is, "I don't know, because it has not been looked at." And in the current climate of containing costs, what we hear is "No. We will not pay, because it is not proven." We're running a risk of stopping progress through this kind of policy, and I'm very concerned about it.

Question: How do you become aware of research results?

Dr. Banta: The most important way is informal, at a conference, or by word of mouth. When Congress asks a question, we look into the literature and have developed quite an institutional memory. After these reviews, we then talk to the experts.

Question: How do you feel the thrust toward competition and decentralization (block grants, for example) will affect policymaking?

Dr. Banta: Since I don't think competition is going to come to anything, I don't think it is going to affect policymaking very much. The broad view is that we have to change the nature of the reimbursement program to make better use of scientific data for decision making. Furthermore, fees will be set at such a level that they won't provide an appropriate incentive for developing technological procedures.

Most programs will remain at the national level. I think there will be a kind of philosophical shift, that is, decisions will be made more at the local level than at the federal level, but I don't see much in the way of formal change toward medical technology itself. And I think the only source of substantial amounts of money for evaluation of technology is the federal budget. I don't think the states, the private sector, or the medical schools are going to come up with it.

State Policy Interviews— Medical Technology Decision Making: A Telephone Survey

Paul M. Allen

Director of Medical Services Administration
Michigan Department of Social Services
Lansing, MI

Question: What types of policy decisions does your department make?

Mr. Allen: We establish policy on the type of services that the state will pay for and the scope of health services that beneficiaries may require at the expense of the Medicaid program. We are the Medicaid agency for the state, so our decisions encompass the whole range of Medicaid coverage for the state of Michigan.

Question: How do you set policy on medical technology?

Mr. Allen: Medical technology is usually developed in the marketplace by the health care industry. We become aware of new developments as we provide and pay for health benefits. As a new technology matures, we are usually approached by the developer to provide benefit coverage for it. We don't usually go out and research new developments ourselves.

Question: What steps must occur in the decision-making process?

Mr. Allen: We have a group that is concerned with Medicaid policy and coverage. The members study various aspects of coverage and become familiar with new technologies such as CAT scanners, as they can be applied to neonatal coverage or the special needs of disabled or geriatric patients. The actual coverage decision is based on an informal consensus of managers and health care analysts that a certain service is desirable and that funds are in fact available to pay for it: that it is worth the money. That's always the bottom line: Does the procedure solve a preventive or life-threatening problem? Does it provide better health care? Is it cost effective? We usually draft a policy statement on a new issue—whether a procedure or technology should qualify as a covered benefit, for instance— and we circulate it among our own medical staff as well as consultants who work with us: MDs, osteopaths, laboratories, physical therapists, and so on. Decisions on drugs are a classic example of this procedure.

Question: What problems do you face in establishing new policies?

Mr. Allen: With most new medical technology there is no consensus as to its worth. A developer suggests we cover a certain device or product, and we immediately have a conflict. Some people may say it isn't worth anything, others may say it's marginal, while a third group claims it's the greatest thing since sliced bread! These early reports are subjective. We try to get a consensus from the professionals who prescribe the drug or use the instrument and evaluate the results. Again, the issue is whether the budget can afford it after an informed group has agreed that it is a good idea.

Question: Who are the key participants in the total process?

Mr. Allen: They are a combination of the external public, internal activists, and lobbyists. Also, the opinions of consultants weigh heavily on the decision-making process.

Question: Where do you fit in?

Mr. Allen: As the director of the Medicaid agency that makes these decisions, I am responsible for the decisions after others have made suggestions.

Question: How do you assess the costs, risks, and benefits of a medical technology?

Mr. Allen: We try to determine from the opinions of health professionals whether a new technology can prolong life, prevent major illness, or provide insurance against life-threatening situations.

Question: What factors are addressed in this process?

Mr. Allen: We find out to what extent this new technology will benefit the total population and ultimately improve health. We then quantify costs vs benefits; we find out what it would cost to implement. Then we decide whether the budget can afford it.

Question: How might research results aid your decision-making?

Mr. Allen: Research results add another body of opinion. The problem with research, of course, is that it's often conducted by partial observers who want to see a certain outcome. We need to separate truth from bias. The problem is that it's very difficult if not impossible to be completely objective. This problem is implicit in a process like the one I've described, where industry and innovators necessarily have more information than we have on the item they are trying to sell. There is no cure for subjectivity. All we can do is try to research the use of the product in a more objective situation.

Question: How do you become aware of research results?

Mr. Allen: Most often, someone approaches us with a product—salespeople, public relations, research staff—someone employed by the producers. There is some input from journals, but not much.

Question: How will the thrust towards competition and decentralization—block grants, for example—affect policy-making?

Mr. Allen: It will shift the scene of activity from the national level to the state level. I hope it will make the distribution of funds and effort more responsive to community needs. It's hard to knock the concept that the people who provide the resources should know how to spend them. In many places, the tax dollars and financing come from a local source, and perhaps local people in their wisdom might be able to make some of the decisions. The people in Washington aren't omniscient; they don't know more about what might be needed here than the people of Michigan, but again, some of the local people don't have access to all the information they might need to make a decision. However, that's a danger inherent in any decision-making process.

State Policy Interviews — Medical Technology Decision Making: A Telephone Survey

Clifton A. Cole, M.P.A.

Chief Deputy Director for Medical Care Services
California Department of Health Services
Sacramento, CA

Question: What types of policy decisions does your department make?

Mr. Cole: All medical and administrative policy decisions related to medical services and the nature and amount of payments in the Medicaid program for services provided.

Question: How is policy concerning medical technology set?

Mr. Cole: There are several different inputs to the policy-making level. The most frequent is by feedback from the field, through the appeal process, and through observations of the consultant personnel reviewing requests for treatment from providers of service. When policies are not in line with general practice in the community, they are challenged through the appeal process: first there is a denial of payment, and that denial is appealed by the provider of care. If the appeal involves a new technique or methodology, evidence for it is presented at the appeals hearing by the provider of care. The appeals are reviewed by the policy staff, which decides whether to recommend a change in policy to the director, who decides whether to approve or disapprove the change in policy.

Another way that policy is determined is by hearings on applications for new policy. For example, we have a Medical Therapeutic and Technical Advisory Committee. Various manufacturers or distributors of drugs apply to have their products included in the drug formulary, or to have their new technique or medical equipment and supplies adopted by the department. The applications are heard in an open, public hearing. All the evidence, pro and con, on the change is aired, and a hearing officer makes a recommendation to the department on whether to adopt, change, or modify the policy. Meanwhile, the staff goes over the recommendation, looks at the pros and cons, and adds information if necessary. This recommendation is then presented to the director, who decides whether to change the policy.

A third way that policy is made involves the legislature. Many times pressure groups—lobbyists or what have you—make requests in the legislature on behalf of their clients and a legislative bill is proposed. The administration must testify whether we support or oppose it. If the administration opposes it, then the department must present testimony against it. If the department supports it, then of course there is no need for further testimony. If the law is passed, the resultant policy is determined by the intent of the law, and the department responds by developing regulations to implement that policy.

Question: What problems do you face in trying to establish new policies?

Mr. Cole: Sometimes the department finds that it needs statutes amended or a new statute to change a policy. Then, if the providers and the people affected by the policy object to it, once again we have a legislative hearing. The objectors present testimony, and the department has to defend itself. Many times lobbyists and other pressure groups are barriers to progress in the direction that the department wants to go. We sometimes have to drop everything to go work up a case against the proposed legislation or substitute a policy more acceptable.

"

Other problems concerning policy are internal. The technical staff may have to work with a policy that they are not in favor of.

Question: Who are the key actors involved in the total process?

Mr. Cole: The legislators, public, lobbyists, health care providers, and our own department, which may include the Governor's office and Department of Finance.

Question: Where do you fit in this process?

Mr. Cole: I am on the director's staff as the chief deputy director for medical care. My basic responsibility is operations, not policy determination. The health care policy for this department is established by a separate division, the Health Care Policy and Standards Division. I mainly implement their determinations. However, much input to that Division's determinations comes from the operations and program staff. Implementing the policy is generally not as difficult as setting it. Most of the time, the mechanisms are already established. Changes are made by internal instruction—by memorandum, by training and orientation—of the people who will carry out the policy. I work with the staff to devise the methodology for implementation and provide feedback to policy formulation staff.

Question: What factors do you address in the process?

Mr. Cole: Right now, under our austerity program, the major factor is cost containment. We usually derive a cost-benefit ratio for any new policy implementation by estimating the number of people it will take to implement and the cost versus the cost savings or other benefits that will result from it.

Question: How are research results used to aid your decision making?

Mr. Cole: If you consider experience as research, then the experience we've had with a similar situation, or the experience we've gathered from small surveys plays a very important part. We also go to the field offices to research the number of requests for a change in policy. So the type of research is important although it may not be scientific.

Question: How does current research not meet your needs? How could it be improved?

Mr. Cole: The cost of doing research and the time required is too great in relation to the importance of getting the policy implemented, particularly for cost containment purposes. Those needs are more immediate. Research and planning for us is a luxury. However, we have built up quite a backlog of experience and evaluation which lends itself to limited research.

Question: How do you become aware of research results?

Mr. Cole: Some research projects are done under contract for the department. We have an internal statistical section, and research component, the Center for Health Services Research and Statistics. We also use our own files—our paid claims tapes— to determine the frequency of use of certain modalities. Most of the research is based on internal records and history files in our computer data bank.

Question: How will the thrust towards competition and decentralization—block grants, for instance—affect policy making?

Mr. Cole: In the past the federal grants process was a direct relationship between the recipient or grantee and the federal government. As a result, the state in the past has not been involved. The way they are currently proposed to be given to the states will not come under my jurisdiction. The legislature will not likely decide to what extent the state will participate and if we do it will be under another section or department.

APPENDIX E

Select Terms Pertaining to Ulcer Disease and CBA/CEA

Select Terms Pertaining to Ulcer Disease and CBA/CEA

Antacid - Any agent that reduces or neutralizes acidity, as of the gastric juice.

Average daily census - The average number of inpatients within a facility each day for a given time period.

Betazole - Stimulant used for gastric acid secretion testing. Betazole possesses less of the undesired side effects of histamine and does not require the concomitant administration of an antihistamine.

Capitation financing method - The method of paying for medical care on a fixed, periodic prepayment basis per individual enrolled in a health plan. Payment by "capitation" implies that the amount paid by the individual is independent of the number of services that individual has received.

CEA/CBA - A composite term referring to a family of analytical techniques that are employed to compare costs and benefits of programs or technologies. Literally, the term as used in this assessment means "cost-effectiveness analysis/cost-benefit analysis."

Cephalic phase - First phase of gastric secretion; represents the secreting response to the sight, smell, taste, and anticipation of food. Mediated by the vagus nerve which in turn leads to acid secretion by direct stimulation of parietal cells in the stomach and by an increased release of gastrin.

Chronic ulcer - A longstanding ulcer with fibrous scar tissue in the floor of the ulcer (can also refer to an ulcer in which the lesion is not that deep).

Cimetidine - H_2 receptor antagonist that has been used successfully in the medical treatment of patients with ulcer disease.

Controlled clinical trial - An experimental design which assigns human or animal subjects, in accordance with predetermined rules, either to an experimental group (in which subjects receive a clinical intervention or dosage level of uncertain efficacy or safety) or to a control group (in which subjects receive some other intervention or dosage level, usually the customary or conventional one, or a placebo). If the predetermined rules specify that the subjects are assigned to groups randomly, the result is a randomized controlled clinical trial.

Cost-benefit analysis - An analytical technique that compares the costs of a project or technological application with the resultant benefits, with both costs and benefits expressed by the same measure. This measure is nearly always monetary.

Cost-effectiveness analysis - An analytical technique that compares the costs of a project or of alternative projects with the resultant benefits, with cost and benefits/effectiveness not expressed by the same measure. Costs are usually expressed in dollars, but benefits/effectiveness are ordinarily expressed in terms such as "lives saved," "disability avoided," "quality-adjusted life years (QALYs) saved," or any other relevant objectives. Also, when benefits/effectiveness are difficult to express in a common metric, they may be presented as an "array."

Criterion variable - An evaluative standard which can be used to measure a program's or program component's performance or effect.

Device (medical) - Any physical item, excluding drugs, used in medical care (including instruments, apparatus, machines, implants, and reagents).

Direct cost - A cost identifiable with a specific program activity.

Discount rate - A factor used in economic analysis to reduce to present value those costs and effects that will occur in future years. Discounting is based on two premises: 1) individuals prefer to receive benefits today rather than in the future, and 2) resources invested today in alternative programs could earn a return over time.

Duodenal ulcer - Ulcer of the duodenum; most usual location of peptic ulcer.

Duodenitis - Inflammation of the duodenum.

Duodenoscopy - Observation of the interior of the duodenum by means of an endoscope.

Duodenum - The first division of the small intestine, about 11 inches in length.

Drug - Any chemical or biological substance that may be applied to, ingested by, or injected into humans in order to prevent, treat, or diagnose disease or other medical conditions.

Economic feasibility - Evaluation of a program's potential for success based on factors such as construction and equipment costs, revenue sources, service costs, and population economic indicators.

Effectiveness - Same as efficacy (see below) except it refers to "…average conditions of use."

Effectiveness measures - Criterion variables which measure the extent to which the goals and objectives of the program in question are being met and the impact of that program.

Efficacy - The probability of benefit to individuals in a defined population from a medical technology applied for a given medical problem under ideal conditions of use.

Endoscope - Instrument used to examine the interior of a canal or hollow organ.

Erosion - Circumscribed defect which involves only the most superficial layer of tissue.

Fee-for-service - A method of paying for medical care by which each service actually received by an individual bears a related charge.

Gastric phase - Second phase of gastric secretion; induced by the presence of food in the stomach; it involves stimulation of chemical receptors in the gastric wall.

Gastric ulcer - Ulcer located in the stomach.

H₂ receptor antagonists - Drugs which inhibit basal acid secretion and secreting responses to feeding, gastric, histamine and vagal stimulation.

Health services research - A field of inquiry that focuses on the structure, production, distribution, and effects of delivering personal health services.

Health system indicators - Measurements of health system performance in delivery of services. Health system indicators are explicit measures of broad qualities (eg, accessibility, continuity and productivity).

Histamine - Powerful stimulant of gastric secretion and constrictor of bronchial smooth muscle.

Human capital - An economic concept used to assess "livelihood," or the earnings potential of an individual. It has often been used as a proxy for the value of life in terms of an individual's productive capacity to society.

Hydrochloric acid-HCl - The acid of gastric juice.

Indirect cost - A cost which cannot be identified directly with a particular activity, service or product of the program experiencing the cost.

Intestinal phase - Third and final stage of gastric secretion; intestinal phase is due to the entry into or presence of food in the small intestine.

Investigational new drug (IND) application - Abbreviation for "notice of claimed investigational exemption for a new drug." An IND application is submitted to FDA by a drug's sponsor. It is a request for permission to use the drug in humans in order to investigate the drug's safety and efficacy for specific conditions. It must include the results of toxicity studies in animals, the qualifications of the investigators, and the design of the proposed clinical studies.

Life costs - Mortality, morbidity, and suffering associated with a given medical procedure or disease. Life costs of diagnosis and therapy may be contrasted with their financial costs, the money required for their provision. Life costs of treating a disease can be compared with the mortality, morbidity, and suffering (life costs) resulting from the untreated disease while financial costs are compared with the various monetary costs of not treating the disease. Use of life costs in assessing the costs of medical procedures avoids the need for assigning dollar values to mortality and morbidity.

Marginal benefit - An economic concept referring to the additional benefit achieved by incurring an additional unit of cost.

Marginal cost - An economic concept referring to the additional cost of achieving one more unit of benefit.

Medical technology - The drugs, devices, and medical and surgical procedures used in medical care, and the organizational and support systems within which such care is provided.

Morbidity - Illness, injury, impairment, or disability in an individual.

Mortality - The death of an individual; often used in epidemiological studies where death rates for a population for a certain disease or injury are calculated.

Mucosa - Mucous membrane.

Net cost analysis - A form of CEA/CBA (see above) that concentrates on costs, with less attention paid to analyzing outcomes in terms of health benefit. When alternatives are under study, their efficacy is often assumed to be equal.

New drug application (NDA) - An application to the FDA by the sponsor of a new drug for permission to market the drug. The NDA must provide information that demonstrates the safety and efficacy of the drug.

Opportunity cost - In health economics, the value that resources would have if used to the best advantage. When opportunity costs exceed the value of the resources in the way they are being used, they represent lost opportunities to gain value from the resources. Opportunity costs are the appropriate cost concept to consider when making resource allocation decisions. Actual costs, often but not always, can be assumed to represent opportunity costs.

Parietal cells - Stomach cells which secrete hydrochloric acid.

Penetrating ulcer - An ulcer extending into the deep layers beneath the surface of an organ.

Pepsin - A digestive enzyme (protease) of the gastric juices.

Peptic ulcer - An ulcer located in the stomach or duodenum.

Per diem rate - Institutional costs per day of care.

Perforated ulcer - Ulcer extending through the wall of an organ.

Productivity measures - Measures which relate the output of an organization to the input required to produce the product or activity. The ratio indicates how efficiently the product or service is being provided.

Program evaluation - Systematic examination of a specific program to obtain decision-making information on the program's products or services and its short- and long-term productivity.

Proportionate mortality rate - A measure which tells the relative importance of a specific cause of death in relation to all deaths in a population group.

$$PMR = \frac{\text{number of deaths from a given cause in a specific period of time}}{\text{total deaths from the same time period}} \times 100$$

Pyloric stenosis – Narrowing of the gastric outlet especially by congenital muscular thickening and scarring from previous peptic ulcer.

Pylorus - The muscular tissue surrounding and controlling the outlet of the stomach.

Quality-adjusted life year (QALY) - A health status index in which 1 year of life is adjusted for various types and degrees of disability to yield 1 year of healthy life. QALYs are sometimes used to measure in common terms the effects on morbidity and mortality of health care technologies or programs.

Relative value scale - A coded listing of physician or other professional services using units which indicate the relative value of the various services performed, taking into account the time, skill and overhead cost required for each service, but not usually considering the relative cost-effectiveness of the services, the relative need or demand for them, or their importance to people's health.

Risk - A measure of the probability of an adverse or untoward outcome's occurring. The severity of the resultant harm to health of individuals in a defined population associated with use of a medical technology applied for a given medical problem under specified conditions of use.

Risk-benefit analysis - The formal comparison of the probability and level of adverse or untoward outcomes versus positive outcomes for any given action. The comparison of outcomes does not take into consideration the resource costs involved in the intended action.

Safety - A judgment of the acceptability of risk (see above) in a specified situation.

Standardized mortality ratio (SMR) -Comparison of the expected deaths obtained with the number actually observed in the smaller population.

Tagamet® - Brand name for cimetidine; drug produced by SK&F

Ulcer - A lesion on the surface of the skin or mucous surface, caused by superficial loss of tissue, usually with inflammation.

Vagotomy - Operation in which the vagus nerve is cut.

Vagus nerve - Cranial nerve which, among other functions, influences gastric acid secretion.

Willingness-to-pay - An economic concept used to assess the monetary value of life in terms of what an individual is "willing to pay" to prolong life or postpone death. The willingness-to-pay technique is used to try to assess how much an individual values his or her own life. Sometimes, the technique is also used to assess how much an individual is willing to pay to decrease risk to others or to prolong others' lives.

Zollinger-Ellison syndrome - A clinical condition marked by peptic ulceration with gastric hypersecretion of acid and a particular type of tumor in the pancreas.

REFERENCES

1. Bardhan KD: *Duodenal ulcer: A Current Medical Perspective,* Philadelphia, Smith Kline Corporation, 1978

2. Blalock H Jr: *Social Statistics.* New York, McGraw-Hill Book Company, 1976

3. Boyd WP, Boyce HN: Diagnosis and management of duodenal ulcer disease. *Hospital Medicine* 13: 68–87, 1977

4. Government Studies and Systems. *A Glossary of Health Development Terms.* Contract No. HRA 230-76-0105, Philadelphia, 1976

5. Health Planning Research Services, Inc. Region III Center for Health Planning. *Glossary of Health Terms for Reference.* Contract No. HRA 230-76-0091, DHEW, Fort Washington, PA, 1976

6. McGuigan JE: Peptic ulcer, in Isselbacher KJ et al (eds): *Harrison's Principles Of Internal Medicine,* ed 9. Section 5: Disorders of Alimentary Tract. New York, McGraw-Hill Book Company, 1980, pp 1371–1384

7. National Institute of Arthritis, Metabolism and Digestive Diseases, NIH. Peptic Ulcer, Bethesda, Maryland, 1978

8. Office of Technology Assessment, Congress of the United States. *The Implications of Cost-Effectiveness Analysis of Medical Technology,* August 1980

9. Sellitz C et al: *Research Methods in Social Relations.* New York, Holt, Rinehart and Winston, 1976

10. Staff of the Committee on Interstate and Foreign Commerce, US House of Representatives. *A Discursive Dictionary of Health Care,* GPO No. 052-070-03199-9, 1976

11. *Stedman's Medical Dictionary,* ed 23. The Williams & Wilkins Company, Baltimore, Maryland, 1976.

APPENDIX F

Selected Bibliography

Contents

Cost-Benefit/Cost-Effectiveness Analysis of Health Technology Selected Bibliography

The following bibliography on cost-benefit/cost-effectiveness analysis (CBA/CEA) of health technology consists of recent references selected to provide conference participants with an overview of recent research and discussion pertinent to the symposium, Cost-Benefit and Cost-Effectiveness Analysis in Policy Making: Cimetidine as a Model.

There have been several recent reviews of CBA/CEA in health care, some of which are described on page 1 of this compilation. This bibliography is designed in part to update these works.

In preparing the bibliography the following sources were searched: Medlars, National Library of Medicine Data Bases, 1978–1981; Business Periodicals Index, 1978–1981; National Technical Information: Weekly Government Abstracts on Health Planning and Health Services Research, 1978–1981; and recent issues of pertinent journals. References obtained were reviewed and selections were made that complement the symposium presentations. Therefore, this bibliography should not be considered a comprehensive review of CBA/CEA in health care.

Abstracts are provided when available from sources consulted. No original abstracting was performed.

MAJOR REVIEWS

Hellinger FJ: Cost-benefit analysis of health care: Past applications and future prospects. *Inquiry* 17:204–215, 1980

This paper briefly discusses the general principles of cost-benefit analysis and an analysis of how these techniques have been applied to questions of intervention in the health field is presented. A discussion of how cost-benefit analysis may be extended to the area of health care regulation, and outlines of two cost-benefit studies of specific health care regulations, are also included.

Warner KE, Hutton RC: Cost-benefit and cost-effectiveness analysis in health care: growth and composition of the literature. *Medical Care* 18:1069–1084, 1980

Concern about the escalating costs of health services is reflected in the rapid growth of the literature on cost-benefit and cost-effectiveness analysis in health care. A search of that literature from 1966–1978 produced a bibliography of more than 500 relevant references, growing from half a dozen per year at the beginning of the period to close to 100 during the most recent 2 years. The literature growth has been more rapid in medical than nonmedical journals and a preference for CEA over CBA appears to be emerging. Studies related to diagnosis and treatment have gained in popularity, while the early prominence of studies with a substantive prevention theme have diminished. Consistent with the increasing medical focus of the literature, numbers of articles oriented toward individual practitioner decision making have grown more rapidly than those oriented toward organizational or societal decision making. In addition to documenting these trends, this article identifies published reviews of health care CBA/CEA and books and articles attempting to convey the principles of CBA/CEA to the health care community. The article concludes with speculation on probable near-future trends in the literature and consideration of the quality implications of the rapid growth.

PRINCIPLES OF CBA/CEA

Cost-benefit and cost-effectiveness analysis. [letter] *New England Journal of Medicine* 304:432, 1981

Caper SP: Measuring the efficiency and effectiveness of medicine. *Medical World News* 20:63, 1979

Fuchs VR: What is CBA/CEA, and why are they doing this to us? *New England Journal of Medicine* 303:937–938, 1980

Griffiths DA: Economic evaluation of health services. Concepts and methodology applied to screening programmes. *Revue Épidémiologie Santé Publique* 29:85–101, 1981

This methodological review explains the different levels of economic analyses, the nature and use of which are often not clearly understood. These include analyses of cost productivity, cost effectiveness, and cost benefit. The types of costs to be considered are then identified and classified into four groups according to whether they are direct or indirect, and visible or invisible. A numerical practical example of the cost-effectiveness of a breast cancer screening program is used to demonstrate the techniques used in practice, and the types of problems and questions that may occur. The paper concludes that the development of epidemiological and economic models can make a significant contribution to the analysis of the complex interrelationships that prevail in the health services, and to the identification of crucial aspects for research and decision making concerning intervention strategies.

Kelman S: Cost-Benefit Analysis: An Ethical Critique. *Regulation* 5:33–40, January/February 1980; also in *Across Board* (NY) 18:74–82, July/August 1981

McCarthy NJ: Benefit-cost and cost-effectiveness analysis: Theory and application. *Developments in Biological Standardization* 43:403–417, 1979

Mushkin SJ, Landefeld JS: *Biomedical Research: Cost and Benefits.* Cambridge MA, Ballinger Publishing Co., 1979

Rowe WD: Risk/benefit determination. *American Industrial Hygiene Association Journal* 40:1200–1206, 1979

Shepard DS, Thompson MS: First principles of cost effectiveness analysis in health. *Public Health Report* 94:535–543, 1979

Tait GW: Cost-benefit analysis: Reality or illusion? [letter] *Health Physics* 39:835–838, 1980

Watts CA et al: Cost effectiveness analysis: Some problems of implementation. *Medical Care* 17:430–434, 1979

Cost-benefit analyses in the health sector frequently deal with situations in which the money value of the benefits is either difficult or impossible to measure. This paper asserts that the use of cost-effectiveness analysis as a means of escaping the need to place a dollar value on benefits does not avert the need for appropriately discounting these benefits when they accrue in different periods over time. The choice of an appropriate discount rate is discussed, and the benefits of elective hysterectomy are used to demonstrate that a serious bias can result from ignoring the need for discounting.

150

Weinstein MC, Stason WB: Foundations of cost-effectiveness analysis for health and medical practices. *New England Journal of Medicine* 296:716–721, 1977

The value and application of cost-effectiveness analysis to the health care field are considered, and foundations of the analysis in the allocation of health care resources are described. Prerequisites for useful cost-effectiveness analysis are identified. A distinction is made between cost-effectiveness analysis and cost-benefit analysis in the assessment of health practices. The underlying premise of cost-effectiveness analysis is that, for a given level of available resources, the goal is to maximize total aggregate health benefits. In cost-benefit analysis for a given health benefit goal, the objective is to minimize the cost of achieving it. Elements of cost-effectiveness analysis are noted as the cost-effectiveness ratio, net health care costs, net health effectiveness, the discounting of future costs and health benefits through present value analysis, and sensitivity analysis. It is concluded that the primary advantage of formal cost-effectiveness analysis in the health care field is that it forces one to be explicit in allocation decisions. Equations are provided and a table shows hypothetical programs with varying timing of costs and health benefits.

CBA/CEA AS A DECISION TOOL

Cost-effectiveness Analysis in Health System Planning. Princeton, NJ: Educational Testing Service, 1979. (Available NTIS: HRP-0902010/8)

Concepts in cost effectiveness analysis are outlined in this course to facilitate health system planning. Both cost-effectiveness analysis and health system planning are defined and a distinction is made between cost-effectiveness and other terms frequently used in the literature (cost benefit and cost utility). Instruction includes reasons for the performance of cost-effectiveness analysis, common problems that occur, and strategies for their resolution. Health planners are shown how to calculate the cost effectiveness of an alternative combination of long-range actions or a single action, identify what information is used in planning and the plan development phase from which information is obtained (assessment, goal/need analysis, action design), describe types of costs used in calculating effectiveness, and note assumptions on which cost-effectiveness analysis is based. Sections of the unit pertain to such areas as alternative plans and techniques for refining cost-effectiveness analysis.

Ashford NA: Alternatives to cost-benefit analysis in

regulatory decisions. *Annals of the New York Academy of Science* 363:129–137, 1981

Ashford NA: The limits of cost-benefit analysis in regulatory decisions. *Technology Review* 82:70–72, 1980

Baram MS: The use of cost-benefit analysis in regulatory decision-making is proving harmful to public health. *Annals of the New York Academy of Science* 363:123–128, 1981

Bootman JL et al: Cost-benefit analysis: A research tool for evaluating innovative health programs. *Evaluation and the Health Professions* 2:129–154, 1979

This article reviews the evaluation methodology known as cost-benefit analysis. Studies that have utilized this technique are presented and briefly reviewed. In addition, the closely related technique known as cost-effectiveness analysis (CEA) is described and contrasted with cost-benefit analysis. Several research articles utilizing CEA are described. It is recommended that cost-benefit analysis be used as a mechanism to evaluate innovative health programs. This may be the sole mechanism that will enable health practitioners to cost-justify their innovative services to the federal government and other third party payers.

Buxbaum CB: Cost-benefit analysis: The mystique versus the reality. *Social Service Review* 55:453–471, 1981

Cost-benefit analysis is promoted as a method for making social policy decisions more rational. A review of its goals, procedures, assumptions, and recent applications exposes technological shortcomings and implicit value preferences. If the method is to be useful, it must be balanced by the judgment of decision makers. Consequently, the power of cost-benefit analysis to improve policy decisions depends on the political context. In a conservative environment this analysis provides a rationalization for disinvesting in social welfare. At such times social reformers would be wise to engage in political action and to challenge cost-benefit analysis.

Crandell RW: The use of cost-benefit analysis in regulatory decision-making. *Annals of the New York Academy of Science* 363:99–107, 1981

Dittman DA, Smith KR: *Consideration of Benefits and Costs: A Conceptual Framework for the Health Planner.* Evanston, IL, Northwestern University, Program in Hospital and Health Services Management, 1978. (Available NTIS: HRP-0029183/1WW)

The need for a unified approach to considering benefits and costs when establishing priorities and selecting recommended actions arose with the passage of the National Health Planning and Resources Development Act of 1974. This paper is intended to assist health planners by providing them with a clear understanding of concepts and by presenting a viable frame of reference for matching costs and benefits throughout the planning process. The introductory material discusses factors which limit the ability of the marketplace to optimally allocate health care resources and defines the purpose of planning and of cost-benefit analysis. Attention is also given to the nature of several concepts of particular concern to health planners and health systems agencies (HSAs), including goals and objectives, setting priorities, and recommended evaluation of the relative priorities of an HSA's goals and objectives; and to a taxonomy for categorizing the community's health needs. The discussion which follows, on the use of cost-benefit analysis in setting priorities, considers clarification and measurement of benefits of health programs, including direct, indirect, and intangible benefits, cost determination; cost-benefit analysis and the well-functioning market; prioritization of goals; and criteria for making social decisions. Cost effectiveness is addressed and a figure illustrates the interrelationship between cost-effectiveness analysis and cost-benefit analysis.

Fischhoff B: Cost-benefit analysis: An uncertain guide to public policy. *Annals of the New York Academy of Science* 363:173–188, 1981

Recognition of the uncertainty inherent in social plans has generated a variety of formal approaches to coping with uncertainty. Perhaps the most heavily touted and widely adopted are variants of cost-benefit analysis. Although based on an appealing premise and supported by a sophisticated methodology, these procedures have a number of characteristic limits. One set of limits is imposed by the unavailability of necessary inputs to the analysis. Since neither the values nor the likelihood of many costs and benefits can be assessed by any formal computations, they must be derived by human judgment. Research has shown, however, that probability judgments are often quite unreliable and prone to systematic biases, while judgments of value are highly labile, changing with subtle (and formally irrelevant) shifts in the elicitation procedure. The second set of limits arises when one comes to assess the quality of analyses. There have been few systematic evaluations of formal analyses or attempts to develop a methodology for assessment. Again, one is forced to rely upon judgments which research has shown to be untrustworthy. A third set of limits is the inability of the procedures to address critical issues in the management process they are designed to abet.

Krasny J: A new approach to decision making for health care managers. *Health Management Forum* 1:71–87, 1980

Neuhauser D: Cost effective clinical decision making and the medical care manager. *Hospital and Health Services Administration* 25:55–61, 1980

Weinstein MC: Cost-effectiveness analysis for clinical procedures in oncology. *Bulletin du Cancer* 67:491–500, 1980

The provision of medical care consumes resources, and the resources available for the provision of medical care are limited. Decisions are being made at many levels of the health care system, including providers and fiscal intermediaries, to allocate these resources. Such decisions, however, are often inconsistent with the objective of deriving the maximum health benefits from the resources spent. Many cost-effectiveness and cost-benefit studies have been conducted in order to guide present and future resources allocation decisions. Many analyses have not been accepted by health care decision makers because a critical factor or issue has been omitted. In the attempt to be objective, the analyst may avoid uncertainties or subjective value judgments that often dominate the thinking of the decision maker. The role of the analyst in cost-effectiveness analysis, as in decision analysis for the individual patient, is to clarify and highlight such factors, not to obfuscate them. (In English.)

CBA/CEA HEALTH CARE APPLICATIONS

Cost and technology: The management of technology in health and medical care. *Clinical Engineering* 8:13–15, 1980

The Implications of Cost-Effectiveness Analysis of Medical Technology. Washington, DC: Office of Technology Assessment, August 1980. (Available NTIS: PB80-216864)

The assessment analyzes the feasibility, implications, and usefulness of cost-effectiveness and cost-benefit analysis in health care decision making. Five background papers supplement this main report. The subjects covered include: methodology and literature issues, a psychotherapy case study, a diagnostic X-ray case study, 17 case studies of individual medical technologies and a review of international experience in managing medical technology. The 17 case studies have been issued as separate volumes under the collective title

152

Background Paper No. 2.

Golding AM, Tosey D: The cost of high-technology medicine. *Lancet* 2:195–197, 1980

Gottinger HW: Economic evaluation of effectiveness in health care delivery. *Methods of Information in Medicine* 20:101–109, 1981

Hallstrom A et al: Modeling the effectiveness and cost-effectiveness of an emergency service system. *Social Science and Medicine* 15C:13–17, 1981

Haughton JG: Technology and cost containment: A medical dilemma. *Urban Health* 18:8, 1979

Johns RJ: Technology in medicine: Blessing or curse? *Forum on Medicine* 3:406–410, 1980

Johnson K: A cost analysis method for dentistry. *Journal of Marketing for Professions* 1:10–12, 1980

Lave LB: Economic evaluation of public health programs. *Annual Review of Public Health* 1:225–276, 1980

Nelson W, Swint JM: Cost-benefit analysis of fluoridation in Houston, Texas. *Journal of Public Health Dentistry* 36:88–95, 1976

Most previous cost-benefit analyses of fluoridation programs have been retrospective in approach and have biased their results in favor of fluoridation. This report describes in detail a study which performed a prospective cost-benefit analysis for a city which is not using fluoridation—Houston, Texas—applying the results of past studies of the effects of fluoridation. This study performed a prospective analysis of fluoridating a segment of Houston's water supply and explicitly introduced and evaluated the time pattern of the costs and benefits, since it was shown that neglect of the time structure of the costs and benefits would significantly bias the results. A benefit-cost ratio of 1.51 and a new present value (or social profit of $1,102,970) were found. The results are biased downwards and should be considered the lower bound. Thus the results indicate that an investment in a fluoridation program by the city of Houston would be a socially profitable one.

Rogers PJ et al: Is health promotion cost effective? *Preventive Medicine* 10:324–339, 1981

Ruchlin HS et al: The efficacy of second opinion consultation programs: A cost-benefit perspective. *Medical Care* 20:3–20, 1982

Schoenbaum SC: Cost/effectiveness considerations in clinical trials. *Triangle* 19:103–106, 1980

Terris M: Preventive services and medical care: The costs and benefits of basic change. *Bulletin of the New York Academy of Medicine* 56:180–188, 1980

Applications—Pharmaceuticals, Pharmaceutical Services

McGhann WF et al: Cost-benefit and cost-effectiveness—methodologies for evaluating innovative pharmaceutical services. *American Journal of Hospital Pharmacy* 35:133–140, 1978

Various methodologies for evaluating the cost-effectiveness of innovative pharmaceutical services are considered. Process and outcome measures are explored, and suggested steps in a cost-benefit study are presented. Pharmacy studies using both cost-benefit and cost-effectiveness analysis techniques are appraised. The assumptions upon which cost-benefit analysis is based are enumerated, and supporting equations are given. Cost-benefit analysis compares the monetary cost of a program with its expected benefits measured in dollar terms. In cost-effectiveness analysis, one starts with a set of target results and compares the cost of various ways in which target results can be achieved. The following areas of pharmaceutical services are discussed: ambulatory patient consultation, unit dose drug distribution, drug information services, monitoring drug therapy in acute care and long-term care, parenteral admixture services, patient and therapy responsibilities, patient discharge interviews, patient drug histories and profiles, and personnel substitutions.

Perll M, Hamburger S: A comparison of diazepam and chlordiazepoxide—cost effectiveness in the pharmacy. [letter] *Hospital Pharmacy* 14:560, 1979

Singer K: Relative costs of ticrynafen and thiazides. [letter] *New England Journal of Medicine* 13:301:1346, 1979

Stewart JE: Forces and direction of drug product selection legislation. *Medical Marketing and Media* 14:34–36, 38–39, 1979

pharmaceuticals—cimetidine

Assessment of the Social Benefits Deriving From the Introduction of Cimetidine in Italy. Pavia, Italy: University of Pavia, The Institute of Political Economics Studies

The Effect of Cimetidine on Peptic Ulcer Disease in Rhode Island. Providence, RI: Rhode Island Health Services Research, Inc. December 24, 1980, (revised July 8, 1981)

Impact of Cimetidine on the National Cost of Duodenal Ulcers. Bryn Mawr, PA: Robinson Associates, 1978

Physician investigators experienced in the use of cimetidine for duodenal ulcer were interviewed to develop duodenal ulcer patients' patterns of treatment and response with conventional drug therapy. These physicians then provided estimates of treatment and response with the use of cimetidine. These data were translated into cost estimates for the treatment of duodenal ulcer patients, using data from a Stanford Research Institute study as a reliable source of 1977 national ulcer costs. The results of this analysis indicate that, at the physician investigators' projected national cimetidine usage level of 80% of duodenal ulcer patients, the 1977 national health care costs for duodenal ulcer disease would have been reduced by $650 million—a 29% reduction.

Present Cost of Peptic Ulceration to the Dutch Economy and Possible Impact of Cimetidine on This Cost. Rotterdam, Netherlands: Netherland Economics Institute, 1977

Bodemar G et al: Socioeconomic aspects of treatment with cimetidine in peptic ulcer disease. In: *Further Experience With H₂ Receptor Antagonists in Peptic Ulcer Disease and Progress in Histamine Research.* Proceedings of the Symposium held at Capri, October 19–20, 1979. International Congress Series, No. 521. Princeton, NJ: Excerpta Medica, pp 59–67

Culyer AJ, Maynard AK: Cost-effectiveness of duodenal ulcer treatment. *Social Science and Medicine* 15C:3–11, 1981

This British study compares the costs of treating duodenal ulcer disease with a drug regimen and surgery. A final assessment of the relative advantages of one treatment against the other depends upon the outcome of long-term epidemiological study of the history of the disease with interventions of various kinds. Provisional results indicate that relative costliness per case depends mainly on the scope of the costs considered (eg, institutional or social) and on the rate of discount; taking account of social costs and using the Treasury's public sector discount rate, the use of drugs in suitable cases appears less costly.

Fineberg H, Pearlman L: Cimetidine or surgery for treatment of peptic ulcer? CAHP (Center for the Analysis of Health Practices) *Newsletter* 4:1–5, Spring 1981

Geweke J, Weisbrod B: Some economic consequences of technological advance in medical care: The case of a new drug. In: Helms R (ed): *Drugs and Health-Economic Issues and Policy Objectives.* Washington, DC, American Enterprise Institute for Public Policy Research, 1981, pp 235–272

Hertzman P et al: *The Economic Costs of Ulcer Disease*. Report 1979:6. Lund, Sweden, The Swedish Institute for Health Economics, December 1979, p 72

Muttarini L: A functional view of cost/benefit analysis in peptic ulcer disease. In: *Further Experience With H₂ Receptor Antagonists in Peptic Ulcer Disease and Progress With Histamine Research*. Proceedings of the Symposium held at Capri, October 18–20, 1979. International Congress Series, No. 521. Princeton, NJ, Excerpta Medica, pp 70–82

Oosthuizen H: *Cost of Peptic Ulceration to the South African Economy and the Possible Impact of Tagamet on This Cost*. Prepared for Bureau of Economic Research. Stellenbosch, South Africa, University of Steuenbosch, August 1978

Ricardo-Campbell R et al: Preliminary methodology for controlled cost-benefit study of drug impact: The effect of cimetidine on days of work lost in a short-term trial in duodenal ulcer. *Journal of Clinical Gastroenterology* 2:37–41, 1980

The phase II/III U.S. clinical drug trials for cimetidine (Tagamet®) in duodenal ulcer were examined for their potential application to cost-benefit analysis. Data on "time lost from work" were obtained from a special protocol added to these short-term, double-blind trials of cimetidine. Sixty-four outpatients from the clinical trials remained from an original pool of 217 after exclusion of those subjects who were either retired, unemployed, or of uncertain employment status. Cimetidine was significantly more effective than placebo in reducing "time lost from work" during ulcer disease. The patients' "time lost from work" occurred as a strikingly all-or-nothing phenomenon. We concluded that a prospective clinical trial is appropriate for gathering economic data.

Sonnenberg A, Hefti ML: The cost of postsurgical syndromes (based on the example of duodenal ulcer treatment). *Clinical Gastroenterology* 8:235–247, 1979

von Haunalter G, Chandler VV: *Cost of Ulcer Disease in the United States*. Menlo Park, CA, Stanford Research Institute, 1977

Applications—
Screening/Testing/Diagnosis

Blaine JM: Some thoughts on periodic health screening—examining the physical. *Group Practice Journal* 29:23–26, 1980

Carel RS, Leshem G: Evaluation of the cost-effectiveness of an automated multiphasic health testing system. *Preventive Medicine* 9:689–697, 1980

Clayman CB: Mass screening: Is it cost-effective? [editorial] *Journal of the American Medical Association* 243:2067–2068, 1980

Doberneck RC: Breast biopsy: A study of cost-effectiveness. *Annals of Surgery* 192:152–156, 1980

Farber ME, Finkelstein SN: A cost-benefit analysis of a mandatory premarital rubella-antibody screening program. *New England Journal of Medicine* 300:856–859, 1979

Grande P et al: Optimal diagnosis in acute myocardial infarction: A cost-effectiveness study. *Circulation* 61:723–728, 1980

The predictive value of a diagnostic test estimates the likelihood for presence or absence of disease in a patient with a positive or negative test result. Authors evaluated the predictive values of serum activities of the heart-specific creatine kinase isoenzyme MB (CK-MB), aspartate aminotransferase, lactate dehydrogenase, CK, and ECG in 401 consecutively admitted patients suspected of acute myocardial infarction (AMI). The study showed that CK-MB was better than the other enzymes (single as well as serial) and ECG, evaluated both separately and in combinations. In all cases of AMI, CK-MB was positive within 17 hours after admission. Replacement of the standard enzymes with CK-MB provides a faster and safer diagnosis of AMI and reduces hospitalization time considerably for patients without AMI.

Hull R et al: Cost effectiveness of clinical diagnosis, venography, and noninvasive testing in patients with symptomatic deep-vein thrombosis. *New England Journal of Medicine* 304:1561–1567, 1981

Until the past decade, physicians were content to base therapeutic decisions on the clinical diagnosis of deep-vein thrombosis. Subsequently, numerous studies demonstrated that clinical diagnosis of this condition is nonspecific. Although many now use objective methods to diagnose venous thrombosis, their relative cost and effectiveness have not been adequately studied. We performed a cost-effectiveness analysis of 516 patients with clinically suspected venous thrombosis who were evaluated by clinical diagnosis, venography, and the less invasive combination of impedance plethysmography and leg scanning. We used this analysis to rank these alternative approaches in terms of both cost and effectiveness. The results indicate that clinical diagnosis is cost ineffective. Venography is cost effective and even more so when applied as an outpatient investigation. Impedance plethysmography plus leg scanning is a practical, less invasive alternative to outpatient venography. The cost of inpatient diagnosis is likely to remain the major cost; thus, emphasis should be placed on outpatient diagnostic procedures.

Kristein MM: The economics of screening for colorectal cancer. *Social Science and Medicine,* Medical Economics 14C:275–284, 1980

Leaman DM et al: Assessing the value of mass screening for coronary risks. *Pennsylvania Medicine* 84:29–31, 1981

Showstack JA et al: Evaluating the costs and benefits of a diagnostic technology: The case of upper gastrointestinal endoscopy. *Medical Care* 19:498–509, 1981

Medical technology assessment has been proposed as a way to encourage more appropriate use of medical technologies, which may in turn lower medical care costs. The application to a diagnostic technology of techniques for medical technology assessment is discussed, using upper gastrointestinal endoscopy as an example. Several generic problems are often encountered when performing an assessment of a diagnostic technology. These problems include the need to weigh relatively concrete data on the value of the information gained from the procedure. In the case of upper gastrointestinal endoscopy, data on morbidity (approximately 2 per 1,000 cases), mortality (approximately 1 per 20,000 cases), charges (approximately $290 per procedure) and costs (between $69 and $128 per procedure) are relatively easy to determine. Less easily calculated is the marginal diagnostic gain from endoscopies performed for the wide variety of conditions for which an endoscopy may be indicated. It is concluded that, in the case of diagnostic technologies, technology evaluations may be most useful as a heuristic tool. Because of the difficulty in weighing costs and benefits, however, formal evaluations of diagnostic technologies will probably not contribute to medical care cost containment in the near future.

Straumfjord JV Jr: How cost effective is videomicroscopy? *Pathologist* 33:616–617, 1979

Insisting that videomicroscopy not be viewed as a luxury to be employed only in large educational institutions and only by audiographics departments, the author substantiates his point by documenting what it cost to institute such a system in his own pathology department.

Wallace RM: Current uses of body plethysmography. *Respiratory Therapy* 9:21–24, 1979

screening/testing/diagnosis— CAT scanners

Abrams HL, NcNeil B: Computed tomography— cost and efficacy implications. *American Journal of Roentgenology* 131:81–87, 1978

This paper considers both computed tomography (CT) cost considerations and measures of CT effectiveness. Scanners cost $550,000 to $750,000, with annual operating costs of approximately $300,000 per year per machine. In view of the effect of patient load on costs, planning agencies are emphasizing the intensive utilization of any proposed CT unit and are encouraging a work week in excess of 40 hours. One study showed that the average cost per examination is $167, which is less than the average charge to patients of $226. Criteria for estimating the required number of CT brain scanners are usually based on the number of neurological disorders per year and/or population. The purported impact of CT on financial costs and savings remains controversial because estimates are generally theoretical. Diagnostic CT of the brain has been demonstrated to be useful, but CT bodyscanning's contribution beyond competing imaging techniques has not yet been fully established. CT body scanning is still a diagnostically accurate method whose efficacy will require further documentation. A table presents data on the ratio of head and body CT scanners to total population in eight countries.

Bartlett JR et al: Evaluating cost-effectiveness of diagnostic equipment—the brain scanner case. *British Medical Journal* 2:815–820, 1978

An approach to evaluating the cost of computerized axial tomography (CAT) scanning of the brain is described. It is pointed out that the same approach could also be used to evaluate the cost of other medical equipment. Three aspects of the introduction of any piece of medical equipment are noted. These include: (1) the effect on existing procedures and equipment; (2) the effect on existing services; and (3) the reduction in mortality that occurs as a result of introducing the equipment. A discussion is presented of ways to assess the demand for brain scanning and other neuroradiological procedures. First, the demand on a CAT scanner after installation at one hospital was assessed and demand was calculated throughout the region. Next, the different types of demand were evaluated. Alternative ways to meet the demand were then identified and the cost implications of the alternatives were considered. The option that seemed best for the community was selected and the value of improved treatment was then assessed. Relevant data on Britain's National Health Service are included.

Evens RJ, Jost RG: Utilization of body computed tomography units: In installations with greater than one-and-a-half years' experience. *Radiology* 13:695–698, 1979

Utilization and economic data from body computed tomography (BCT) units with more than 1 1/2 years' experience are compared with data from 1977. The average unit operates 52 hours per week, examining 34 patients. Head studies constitute 55% of examinations, abdominal and pelvic 38%. The total technical cost of examining 35 patients per week is approximately $348,000. Charges have been reduced since 1977 by approximately 5%; the average annual loss is about $77,000. Technical and professional charges are lower in high-volume institutions. Current Medicare maximum allowable charges are below BCT costs and charges. Only 17% of installations meet the national guidelines of 2,500 patient examinations per year.

Evens RG, Jost RG: Utilization of head computed tomography units: In installations with greater than two-and-a-half years' experience. *Radiology* 131:691–693, 1979

Utilization and economic data from head computed tomography (HCT) units providing more than 2 1/2 years' experience are compared with data from installations in 1976. The average unit operates 60 hours per week, examining 63 patients. Nearly half the examinations are "double" studies, requiring about 53 minutes. The annual total technical cost is approximately $383,000. Charges have been reduced since 1976. While technical charges are lower in high-volume institutions, professional charges are higher. The usual charges and expected net revenues are above Medicare maximum allowable charges but most units meet the national guidelines. There is considerable variation in data from individual facilities; a "typical" HCT unit cannot be defined.

Margulis AR: Whitehouse lecture. Radiologic imaging: Changing costs, greater benefits. *American Journal of Roentgenology* 136:657–665, 1981

Stocking B, Morrison SL: *Image and the Reality—A Case-Study of The Impacts of Medical Technology.* New York, NY, Oxford University Press, Inc., 1978

The introduction of high-cost, advanced medical technology requires careful preliminary planning to ascertain the benefits and costs involved. This book studies the use of the computed tomography (CT) whole body scanner in Great Britain as a prototype case. Prior to its introduction, the CT whole body scanner was not carefully studied by the National Health Service (NHS) of Great Britain. When its widespread use was applied for, NHS denied granting funds for its use. Nevertheless, physicians and hospitals arranged for the funding of the machines. Studies since its introduction show that the whole body CT gives no better information than other diagnostic procedures, and since each machine is so costly, the expense is difficult to justify. The role of private gifts to the NHS is examined with the suggestion that areas of acceptable gifts be delimited as well as the interrelationships between industry and medicine and the NHS. The development and use of computed tomography, its probable developments in the future, and its impacts on medicine, are also outlined. An appendix provides a clinical evaluation of CT's effectiveness for different regions of the body.

Wortzman G, Holgate RC: Reappraisal of the cost-effectiveness of computed tomography in a government-sponsored health care system. *Radiology* 130:257–261, 1979

The predicted reduction in hospital expenditures because of computed tomography (CT) use in a neuroscience unit has not been realized. Three areas of savings had been predicted in 1975 for Toronto General Hospital: fewer angiograms and pneumoencephalograms (PEGs); reduction in hospital stay; and reduction in admissions. The number of angiograms and PEGs has been reduced—angiograms by 21% and PEGs by 84%. That has not translated into significantly lower costs, however, because of the fixed costs involved in maintaining the units. In addition, because of the 10-day backlog for CT scans, contrasted with the immediate availability of an angiogram, many angiograms are still being ordered that could be replaced by CT scans. The situation may shortly be alleviated, however, by the addition of four new CT units. The average length of hospital stay for neurological diagnosis has increased by one-half day since the introduction of the CT equipment; this, too, may be due to the long waiting period. The number of admissions has not been reduced for a variety of reasons. It is concluded that it is still possible to reallocate costs within the health care program but that this activity is being curtailed by budgeting policies and restrictions. It is further concluded that the answer involves the proper use of all neuroradiological procedures under the direction and control of the physician, regional health councils, hospital administrators, and the government.

screening/testing/diagnosis—genetics and birth technology

Anatomy of birth technology. *National Journal* 11:959, 1979

Banta HD, Thacker SB: Assessing the costs and benefits of electronic fetal monitoring. *Obstetrical and Gynecology Survey* 34:627–642, 1979

Banta HD, Thacker SB: *Costs and Benefits of Electronic Fetal Monitoring: A Review of the Literature.* Hyattsville, MD, National Center for Health Services Research. (Available NTIS: PB-294 690/3WW)

This report focuses on electronic fetal monitoring (EFM)—a technology that was developed during the 1960s and has rapidly spread into use in clinical obstetrics. The report includes a review of the extensive published literature on EFM and related subjects, as well as original calculations concerning the technique's specificity and sensitivity, predictive value as a diagnostic test, and financial costs associated with its potential risks.

Thompson M, Milunsky A: Policy analysis for prenatal genetic diagnosis. *Public Policy* 27:25–48, 1979

Consideration of the analytic difficulties faced in estimating the benefits and costs of prenatal genetic diagnosis, coupled with a brief review of existing cost-benefit studies, leads to the conclusion that public subsidy of prenatal testing can yield benefits substantially in excess of cost. The practical obstacles to such programs include the attitudes of prospective parents, a lack of knowledge, monetary barriers, inadequately organized medical resources, and the political issue of abortion. Policy analysis can now nevertheless formulate principles and guide immediate actions to improve present utilization of prenatal testing and to facilitate possible future expansion of these diagnostic techniques.

Wright ML, Elsas LJ 2d: Application of benefit-to-cost analysis to an x-linked recessive cardiac and humeroperoneal neuromuscular disease. *American Journal of Medical Genetics* 6:315–329, 1980

Applications—Treatment/Procedures

Clark CG et al: Cost effectiveness in the treatment of gastric cancer. *Clinical Oncology* 6:303–307, 1980

Guess HA: Bernoulli's cost-benefit analysis of smallpox immunization. [letter] *New England Journal of Medicine* 305:347, 1981

Jackson MW et al: Elective hysterectomy—a cost-benefit analysis. *Inquiry* 15:275–280, 1978

In the case of a 30-year-old woman without symptoms, there would be little, if any financial benefit to be gained from an elective hysterectomy. This conclusion was reached in a study of women served by the Seattle (Washington) Prepaid Health Care Project. Costs incurred due to pregnancy, abortion, or morbidity due to contraception were not included in the calculations. Once the annual cost projections were obtained, the stream of expected benefits was discounted from the present value using a rate of return of 3% as well as a 6.5% discount rate. When discounted at a 3% interest rate, the direct benefit of a hysterectomy was set at $1,822; at the 6.5 present rate, it was reduced to $1,240. Since the mean cost of the operation was $1,637, net benefits at both rates would have been small, namely a benefit of $185 and a net cost of $397, respectively. However, it is acknowledged that many indirect costs and intangible factors would influence a woman's decision regarding hysterectomy.

Koplan JP et al: Pertussis vaccine—an analysis of benefits, risks and costs. *New England Journal of Medicine* 301:906–911, 1979

Using decision analysis, authors estimated the benefits, risks and costs of routine childhood immunization against pertussis. Without an immunization program, we predict that there would be a 71-fold increase in cases and an almost fourfold increase in deaths (2.0 to 7.6) per cohort of one million children. With a vaccination program, we predict 0.1 cases of encephalitis associated with pertussis and five cases of post-vaccination encephalitis; without a program, there would be only 2.3 cases of encephalitis associated with pertussis. Community vaccination would reduce the cost related to pertussis by 61%. Our analysis supports continuation of vaccination in routine childhood immunization programs, but suggests the need for more reliable data on complications from the vaccine, further study of the epidemiology of pertussis and development of a less toxic vaccine.

Miller J: Cost analysis documents true cost of operations. *Same Day Surgery* 4:37–41, 1980

Paxinos J et al: Cost of cardiopulmonary resuscitation. *Hospital Forum* 14:569–572, 1979

Bishop JE: Surgeons find heart repair pays for itself. *Wall Street Journal* [Midwest Ed] 60:13, August 29, 1980

Centerwall BS: Cost benefit analysis and heart transplantation. *New England Journal of Medicine* 304:901–903, 1981

Finkler SA: Cost effectiveness of regionalization: Further results on heart surgery. *Health Services Research* 16:325, 1981

Haberman S: Heart transplants: Putting a price on life. *Health and Social Service Journal* 90:877–879, 1980

Widespread interest was recently evoked by publication in the Sunday Times of some calculations by Steven Haberman, senior lecturer in actuarial science at the City University. These showed that heart transplants fell not into the category of conspicuous medical consumption, but into that of sound economic investment. Dr. Haberman has now reworked his figures for the Journal, taking into account more detailed and authoritative information than was previously available. Using the technique of cost-benefit analysis, he shows that apart from any humanitarian considerations, heart transplants actually save the country money.

APPENDIX G

Symposium Participants

Symposium Participants

Synthesizer:

Bernard S. Bloom, Ph.D.
Chief, Health Services Research,
Veterans Administration Medical Center
Research Associate Professor, Department of
Research Medicine, University of Pennsylvania
Medical School
Senior Fellow, Leonard Davis Institute
Philadelphia, Pennsylvania

USE OF CBA/CEA IN POLICYMAKING

Facilitators:

Harvey Fineberg, M.D., Ph.D.
Professor of Health Policy and Management
Center for Analysis of Health Practices
Harvard School of Public Health
Boston, Massachusetts

Duncan Neuhauser, Ph.D.
Professor of Epidemiology and Community
Health
Case Western Reserve University
Cleveland, Ohio

William P. Pierskalla, Ph.D.
Executive Director
Leonard Davis Institute
Philadelphia, Pennsylvania

Participants:

W. Blount Barner III, R.Ph.
Program Specialist, Vendor Drugs
Texas Department of Human Resources
Austin, Texas

Remmert Bulthuis, Ph.D.
Chief, Medical Projects
Netherlands Economic Institute
The Netherlands

Mary Byrnes, Ph.D.
Planning and Evaluation
Health and Human Services
Washington, D.C.

Anthony J. Culyer, Ph.D.
Deputy Director
Institute of Social & Economic Research
University of York, Heslington
York, England

Kenneth F. Finger, Ph.D.
Acting V.P. for Health Affairs
University of Florida
Gainesville, Florida

Richard Gleckler, R.Ph.
Provider Assistance
Department of Public Welfare
Columbus, Ohio

Andrew F. Ippoliti, M.D.
Assistant Professor of Medicine
UCLA Department of Medicine
Center for Health Sciences
Los Angeles, California

Egon Johnson, Ph.D.
Senior Research Associate
Swedish Planning and Rationalization Institute
Stockholm, Sweden

Bengt Jonsson, Ph.D.
The Swedish Institute for Health Economics
Lund, Sweden

Sanford Luger, R.Ph.
Chief, Bureau of Pharmacy Services
State of New Jersey
Department of Human Services
Trenton, New Jersey

Gerard Nelligan, R.Ph.
Senior Consultant Pharmacist
New York State Department of Social Services
Albany, New York

Michael P. O'Donnell, R.Ph.
Drug Program Coordinator, State of Maine
Department of Human Services
Augusta, Maine

Paul R. Perruzzi
Deputy Director
North Carolina Department of Human Resources
Division of Medical Assistance
Raleigh, North Carolina

Rita Ricardo-Campbell, Ph.D.
The Hoover Institution
Stanford University
Stanford, California

Sheldon Rovin, D.D.S., M.S.
Chairman
Dental Care Systems
School of Dental Medicine
University of Pennsylvania
Philadelphia, Pennsylvania

David Schwartzman, Ph.D.
Professor of Economics
Graduate Faculty
The New School for Social Research
New York, New York

William D. Thompson, R.Ph.
Pharmaceutical Consultant
Blue Shield of California
San Francisco, California

Keith Weikel, Ph.D.
President, Friesen International, Inc.
Washington, D.C.

INTEGRATION OF RESEARCH RESULTS WITH EXTERNAL FACTORS IN THE POLICY- AND DECISION-MAKING PROCESS

Facilitators:

James T. Doluisio, Ph.D.
Dean
College of Pharmacy
University of Texas at Austin
Austin, Texas

Joyce C. Lashof, M.D.
Dean
School of Public Health
University of California
Berkeley, California

Myrle A. Myers, R.Ph.
Chief
Pharmacy and Ambulatory Care Service
Division of Medical Assistance
Department of Social Services
Denver, Colorado

Participants:

Peggy A. Alsup, M.D., M.Ph.
Medicaid Medical Director
Department of Public Health
Bureau of Medical Assistance
Nashville, Tennessee

Ted Collins, R.Ph.
Pharmacy Practices Consultant
State of Wisconsin
Bureau of Health Care Financing
Madison, Wisconsin

Thi D. Dao, Ph.D.
Director of Economic Research
Pharmaceutical Manufacturer's Association
Washington, D.C.

Tom R. Dolan, R.Ph.
Pharmacist Consultant
Department of Public Welfare
301 Centennial Mall South
5th floor
Lincoln, Nebraska

Louis J. Kolek, R.Ph.
Director
Pharmacy Relations
Blue Cross of New Jersey
Newark, New Jersey

Joanne H. Levy, M.C.P.
Manager Special Projects
Leonard Davis Institute
Philadelphia, Pennsylvania

The Honorable Tarkey J. Lombardi, Jr.
Chairman
New York State Senate Health Committee
Albany, New York

John A. Pagliarini, R.Ph.
Chief Medical Care Specialist
State of Rhode Island
Cranston, Rhode Island

Morton L. Paterson, Ph.D.
Cost-Benefit Studies Manager
Smith Kline & French Laboratories
Philadelphia, Pennsylvania

Leighton Read, M.D.
Instructor in Medicine
Harvard Medical School
West Roxbury VA Medical Center
Center for the Analysis of Health Practices
Boston, Massachusetts

Harry M. Rosen, Ph.D.
Chairman
Department of Health Care Administrator
Baruch College/Mt. Sinai
New York, New York

John T. Skhal, Pharm.D.
Vice President
Professional Affairs
California Pharmacists Association
Sacramento, California

162

Vernon K. Smith, Ph.D.
Director
Bureau of Medicaid
Michigan Department of Social Services
Lansing, Michigan

Peter Solyom, R.Ph.
Vice President, Director of Pharmacy Operations
Kaiser Permanente Medical Care Program
Los Angeles, California

William B. Stason, M.D., S.M.
Associate Professor
Center for the Analysis of Health Practices
Harvard School of Public Health
Boston, Massachusetts

Brian Strom, M.D., M.Ph.
Assistant Professor
University of Pennsylvania School of Medicine
Philadelphia, Pennsylvania

Walter L. Trudeau, B.M., B.Ch.
University of California
Davis Medical Center
Sacramento, California

Milton C. Weinstein, Ph.D.
Professor of Policy and Decision Sciences
Center for the Analysis of Health Practices
Harvard School of Public Health
Boston, Massachusetts

Roy Wiese, Jr., R.Ph.
Administrator, Operations Division
Texas Department of Human Resources
Austin, Texas

Karen C. Wood, Ph.D.
Senior Regional Medical Associate
Smith Kline & French
Northridge, California

**PRIORITIES FOR FUTURE STUDIES OF
MEDICAL TECHNOLOGY**

Facilitators:
Clifton A. Cole, M.P.A.
Chief Deputy Director
Medical Care Services
Department of Health Services
Sacramento, California

Robert W. Piepho, Ph.D.
Associate Dean
Division of Clinical Programs
University of Colorado
Health Services Center
School of Pharmacy
Denver, Colorado

Paul D. Stolley, M.D., M.Ph.
Professor, Medicine and Research Medicine
University of Pennsylvania
Philadelphia, Pennsylvania

Participants:
Donald M. Berwick, M.D.
Acting Director of Research
Harvard Community Health Plan
Boston, Massachusetts

Arthur E. Cocco, M.D.
Vice President
American College of Gastroenterology
Baltimore, Maryland

John L. Colaizzi, Ph.D.
Dean and Professor
Rutgers
The State University of New Jersey
College of Pharmacy
Piscataway, New Jersey

Joseph E. Concino, R.Ph.
Pharmaceutical Consultant for Policy
State of Pennsylvania
Department of Public Welfare
Harrisburg, Pennsylvania

Col. Keith W. Curtis, USAF, MSC
Deputy Director, OCHAMPUS
Aurora, Colorado

Rinaldo V. DeNuzzo, R.Ph., M.S.
Professor
Albany College of Pharmacy of Union University
Albany, New York

Stanley N. Finklestein, Ph.D.
Associate Professor of Health Management
MIT Sloan School of Management
Boston, Massachusetts

Robert A. Freeman, Ph.D.
The University of Mississippi
School of Pharmacy
University, Mississippi

Urs Gessner
Head, Health Services Research
Center for Public Health
St. Gallen, Switzerland

Robert C. Jones, Ph.D.
Director, Research and Development
Leonard Davis Institute
University of Pennsylvania
Philadelphia, Pennsylvania

Walter McLean, Jr.
Director
Office of Family Services
Health and Human Resources Administration
Baton Rouge, Louisiana

Barbara J. McNeil, M.D., Ph.D.
Associate Professor of Radiology
Harvard Medical School
Brigham and Women's Hospital
Boston, Massachusetts

Luther Parker, R.Ph., C.A.E.
Executive Director
Texas Pharmaceutic Association
Austin, Texas

Charles K. Pierce
Commissioner
Georgia Department of Medical Assistance
Atlanta, Georgia

Sumner Robinson, Ph.D.
Dean
Massachusetts College of Pharmacy
Boston, Massachusetts

Sanford J. Schwartz, M.D.
Director of the Clinical Efficacy Assessment Project
American College of Physicians
Philadelphia, Pennsylvania

The Honorable Paul Starnes
State Representative
Nashville, Tennessee

Ronald Stewart
State Government Relations Manager
Smith Kline & French Laboratories
Philadelphia, Pennsylvania

Judith L. Wagner, Ph.D.
Senior Research Associate
The Urban Institute
Washington, D.C.

INDEX